I0695630

Change Your Story

From pain to purpose

Caylin Brie White

For my Mom, Patricia, who taught me never to
lose faith.

Foreword by Chrissy Rice

Hi, it's Chrissy. You might remember me from *Goldify*. I met Caylin in the heart of 2020, when the world was in chaos, through a real estate transaction. She seemed giddy to start her life in this new home with her little family, but I knew there was something underneath.

I felt an instant connection with her when we were sitting across the closing table, I just knew she was going to be my soul sister. Little did I know that our friendship would be the start of a complete life transformation for both of us.

I watched Caylin go from a *White Claw* chugger to a midday coconut water sipper. She was living in the darkness for years and didn't know how to find the light. Until one day our forces came together and my light helped guide her darkness away and hers, mine.

This didn't happen overnight, of course, this was a gradual process, in fact, it took more than two years. We went on a thyroid-healing journey together and I began to see her slowly release her fears, which then, in turn, released her chronic pain. There were days of crying, belly laughing, and clearing throat chakras. She went through breakthroughs, breakdowns, ah-ha moments, mental clarity transformations, and truly felt what it was like to not be in any pain - for the first time in many, many years.

It wasn't an easy process for her, and there were days she wanted to give up.

On those days we dug deep to find her superpowers, to coach her through, to find the light. Now, our lights guide each other on this journey, when one goes dim the other one lights the way.

Get ready for the beautiful unfolding of Caylin Brie.

Love and light,
Chrissy

Changing is healing

This book found you.

If this book found its way to you, you may have been called to change your story. It doesn't mean you're broken, you're just needing a change. I'm just here to tell you that you have the power to change your story.

Change Your Story

Throughout this book, you will find interactive ways to change your own story. I encourage you to read this book alongside journaling your free association thoughts, as this is a big part of the healing process. I encourage you to have an open mind and an open heart. And no matter what you believe in, you must believe in yourself.

#ChangeYourStory

As you read and your story begins to change, it's a sign to share your healing journey with others. Inspire others with your own journey with the #ChangeYourStory hashtag.

Guided Change Your Story Meditations

Get your Change Your Story guided meditations, breath work, and energy healing sessions FREE at www.youtube.com/@cbcinked

Introduction

"You've always had the power my dear, you just had to learn it yourself." - Glinda The Good Witch, The Wizard of Oz

The beautiful unfoldment.

Thank you for taking the time to invest in your health. At one point in my life, I did not. And that suffering led me to my own spiritual enlightenment.

Chronic pain plagued my life for 30+ years until one day it finally didn't. This is my story from lifelong pain to spiritual freedom.

This is a journal filled with all the things I tried — spiritually, energetically, physically, and emotionally —to heal myself, the life lessons I learned, and ways to handle real pain. It's everything that worked and didn't work, to connect my mind, body, and soul. It's a hurricane of emotions and raw feelings.
My hope is that you take the gems you read in this book and it changes your story —wherever it is needed most.

I bare my soul in this book by journaling various phases of my pain and healing. I was on a mission to heal a life sentence of chronic pain. I tried literally everything — and I mean everything — from Ashwagandha to hypnosis, I've tried it. And, you'll get to hear it all.

I share the pain journey physically and mentally, no sugar coating, in all of its authentic glory. It gets ugly and dark.

And that darkness showed me exactly how to get to the light.

I am not a physician, nor am I certified to tell you how to eat, live or act. That is not what we are here to do together, dear reader, we are here to learn and heal in our own ways.

Keep reading if you want to heal your life, build a strategy against pain and become the strongest you, yet.

In this book, you'll learn how chronic pain comes to be, where it lives in the body, what that means for your energy, and how to move through it with joy and gratitude. Yes, you will be grateful for your pain by the end of this book.

Thank you for coming along on this journey with me. It will be filled with shocking revelations, grab-a-tissue tears, and a life-changing strategy to grow through the pain. There's no turning back now.

After reading this book, you may never be the same.

Welcome to the wild world of Caylin's chronic pain journey. Ready? I wasn't either.

—

A disclaimer on faith. Throughout this book, I refer to God, Divine, and Source - all one in the same. Please know that I am a believer in God, you can choose to interpret this however you see fit.

I believe angels are always with us. My Dad sent me this prayer when I needed to hear it most. Maybe it will help you today.

Lord, make me an instrument of your peace
Where there is hatred, let me sow love
Where there is an injury, pardon
Where there is doubt, faith
Where there is despair, hope
Where there is darkness, light
And where there is sadness, joy
O Divine Master, grant that I may
Not so much seek to be consoled as to console
To be understood, as to understand
To be loved, as to love
For it is in giving that we receive
And it's in pardoning that we are pardoned
And it is in dying that we are born to Eternal Life
Amen

Laughing through the pain

"A laugh can be a very powerful thing. Why, sometimes in life, it's the only weapon we have." - Roger Rabbit, Who Framed Roger Rabbit?

This is not a love story.

Pain is my life's work. My masterpiece.

I lived in chronic pain — throughout my whole body — for most of my life. I was told it was a lifelong condition.

What I learned, however, is that we have the power to heal ourself. And I found a way.

As a child, I was just like anyone else — running through the woods barefoot until sunset. I was raised in the 1980s, when microwaves provided dinner and we didn't know what we didn't know. I was young and free to figure out who I was until *BOOM*, I hit 10 years old and the headaches started, the back aches, the knee aches, the cracking jaw, the disjointed neck, the rib pain, the separated hips, the sacrum sciatica, the gut problems, the chronic joint pain, the thinning hair — the entire unharmonious lot of it. This was my life 24/7. Just livin' the dream.

I couldn't seem to keep my body together.

No one talks about the mindset of someone who lives in pain, daily. You don't want to do anything, anywhere, with anyone, but you still have to — life doesn't care if you're in pain. All the time, go go go. And you have to be in a good mood and smile through the pain. It's just the way of life. And so, for the better part of three decades, I did just that.

I laughed through the pain.

I spent many, many hours in doctor's offices and hospitals. I've had hundreds of X-rays, ultrasounds, MRIs, bloodwork after bloodwork after bloodwork, and stool and saliva samples. I even refrigerated my pee in a jug for a week. I had so much bloodwork drawn, I thought I was going to get track marks. I checked my temperature every day for five straight years, tracking, measuring, and evaluating. You want lab work? I've got plenty.

It drained my soul.

I can't imagine the amount of money I spent on trying to "fix" myself. I would latch on to the latest phases or health trends, thinking this would be the thing that fixed me.

Pain became my puppeteer.

My mind was riddled with anxiety, waking up in crippling fear most mornings, wondering what type of pain it would be today — low roar, dull aches, or full throttle pounding? It became my schedule, my calendar, and my decision-making power — and it eventually took over my life.

When I turned 37, I was diagnosed with autoimmune, Hashimoto's thyroid disease, Irritable Bowl Syndrome, with gut microbiome levels off the charts, a chronic ligament disorder (whatever that is), and had a 2.7-millimeter calcified thyroid nodule that was extremely high-risk. I cannot tell you how scared I was when the doctor said it had a high potential of being cancerous. That *c-word* is a mental death sentence. I couldn't move without being in pain.

God was saying, *Caylin, it's time to stop partying*. And yet, I didn't.

The self-sabotage years followed because, after a while, you just say screw it and lean in. I numbed the pain with everything you can think of, and that, of course, made it all ten times worse. The problem with that is… everything. It snowballs into poor health, poor mindset, and poor decisions. It affects your relationships, your finances, and your future. My dark night of the soul lasted a lot longer than some — and yet, I was still laughing. My mask.

And because I didn't listen, God turned up the volume.

Over the span of three months, my pain got worse, my little family fell apart, I moved away from decades of friendships, I lost my Dad, I lost my job, and I lost my best friend from kindergarten. I'm actually surprised I didn't lose my hair.

And that's when God offered me what I needed most. **Clarity**.

That's when I started the journey to heal. I was determined to beat this — whatever it was. I was not going to get cancer. I was going to fight it with everything I had, which wasn't much. But I am a born self-learner, and I was determined. Besides, there were people that healed every day, right? Why couldn't I be one of them?

The healing journey is a long one and doesn't ever really end. It's always evolving but there are many beautiful phases of it that are quite magical. And so that's what needed to happen in order for me to heal, I needed to become open to the magic. And, in my case, I needed to be cracked wide open.

I finally started to listen. *Ok, God, I get it. It's time.*

I look back on those years now as a heartfelt lesson of self-awareness. It took years for me to truly surrender. But the moment I did, everything changed.

Change Your Story

- *What are you laughing through right now?*
- *Have you been or do you need to be cracked wide open?*
- *Are you in physical pain?*

Want to help and inspire others? Share your answers with hashtag #ChangeYourStory

Just my daily dose of chronic pain

"Life is pain, Highness. Anyone who says differently is selling something." - Westley, The Princess Bride

I was in my own way.

I've had so many people ask me, what kind of pain are you in, exactly? Can you describe it for me?

It's hard to explain. It's mystery pain, just about everywhere. I'm not talking about a little ache here and there when we get older, I'm talking about full-body tissue damage.

Being diagnosed with a chronic ligament disorder was a fun one. Ehlers Danlos Syndrome, maybe? Have you heard of it? That's the gloss-over with auto-immune. They throw it under any category when they don't quite know what you have wrong with you…

Regardless, after many nights of crying about it, I refused to be my diagnosis.

Defining pain can be tricky. Chronic pain lasts for three months, three years, or three decades. The pain can be there all the time, or it can come and go. It can happen anywhere in your body, at any time. It can be sharp or dull, stabbing or aching. It can happen when you least expect it. It can happen when you're ignoring your body or paying attention to it. It can happen when you are out of balance with your diet. And, it can also happen when everything is going just right.

This type of pain interferes with daily activities, work, social life, relationships, and happiness. It can lead to difficulty thinking, loss of sleep, anxious thoughts, and deep depression which can make your pain worse. This creates a cycle that's incredibly difficult to break. This pain lives with you, it's a part of you.

And, it thrives on fear.

People also ask me, what's the difference between chronic pain and other (normalized) pain? Chronic pain is consistent and often connected to your mind (and energy). It's regular. And normalized pain typically goes away after a while. Take back pain, for instance, it may go away after a few days. Nope, not this. My bones just moved fluidly in my body — in and out of place, causing major inflammation of the joints and a ton of pain.

And when you're in pain, that's all you can think about.

Acute pain, which will happen on top of chronic pain, happens when you get injured, such as experiencing a bruise or a broken bone. You can fully heal from acute pain, and it goes away with treatment — mostly. I had that too. Of course I did, everyone has injuries. In contrast, chronic pain shows up as mysterious, phantom aches that continue long after you recover from any injury or illness. And, yup, you guessed it, it doesn't go away.

The key word here is normalized. We normalize our daily aches and pains as part of growing older. In actuality, our bodies want to be in total health and the pain is a message from your body to make a change. I encourage you to listen to the communication your body is trying to tell you. I didn't for years and paid the price. The good news is that I was stronger than I thought I was.

Spoiler alert: I was the reason for my own pain.

The truth is, I was in my own way. Hi. It's me. I'm the problem, it's me. But I found I was also the solution. We are all our own worst enemies *and* our saving grace. We are the ones who will drag ourselves down to the depths of hell. And, we are the only ones who will save us.

Change Your Story

- *Are you ignoring important pain messages from your body?*
- *Have you normalized something in your life that needs your attention, or perhaps needs to be changed?*
- *Are you in the dark night of the soul or have you suffered enough?*

Root canal revelations

"Just when I think you couldn't possibly be any dumber, you go and do something like this... and totally redeem yourself." - Harry, Dumb and Dumber

Nothing quite like breaking down in the dentist chair.

What if I told you that it took me getting laughing gas during a root canal to truly relax? Well, that happened to me and it may have been my breaking point.

I was living in all different kinds of pain, as you've read, but at this time in my life, I was in tooth pain. If you've ever experienced the pain at the root of a tooth, you know you can't do much else. It runs the show.

During this time, my husband and I were grieving, our little family was torn apart, we were moving homes, leaving friendships, and at our wit's end. It wasn't our finest hour, and our lives were being uprooted without our permission. We were pretending everything was fine and that we were in control. **But the truth of it was that we just needed to let go, but we didn't know how.**

I was in severe 10 out of 10 tooth pain for weeks and the mental anguish was making it worse. One morning, I couldn't handle it anymore and I made an emergency visit to a dentist (I randomly picked one that could take me) and drove off, white-knuckling it. I was in so much pain I couldn't open my mouth to greet the front desk lady. I just started crying, right there in the waiting room. She took one look at me and rushed me back to the chair.

The kindness of these strangers will never be forgotten.

A wonderful team of angels assembled and the dentist whipped around in her chair and said, "Ma'am this is going to be an emergency root canal." Only one of my worst dental fears. I told her to do whatever needed to be done to stop this immense pain and I sat back in the chair with pure fear in my heart. Of course, I'd heard nightmares of root canals and the pain they caused - but nothing could be worse than this.

As the lady reached for the nitrous oxide she asked if I've ever had it before. I said I couldn't remember, it had probably been decades. She said, "Don't worry, it's very relaxing." Well, that's all it took for me, I gladly grabbed the mask because I hadn't been relaxed in years.

And when the slow leak of the gas entered my system, a tear ran down my face as I realized I hadn't breathed or relaxed or taken *one moment* for myself for as long as I could remember. The room went fuzzy and I engulfed myself in total surrender. I

allowed myself to breathe and truly trust for the first
time in forever.

It was a sad but purposeful revelation.

Not only did the root canal go smoothly, but she also
stopped the searing root pain that was currently
plaguing me and I was able to finally breathe. As we
joked about the relaxation and took funny photos
together, I reveled in the laughter of strangers. I
longed for joyous moments that weren't filled with
sadness or regret. It took a root canal to get me to this
point – what a mess.

And, what did I learn?

One, take care of your teeth, which I do! Raised with
a dentist in the family, it was top priority. The dentist,
however, said that this root canal was 'trauma from
my youth' and that really stuck with me. (See my
other book *Goldify* for some explanations, there.) We
hold things in our bodies that we really do need to
release.

And, two, making time for yourself is not optional. It
is mandatory for your sanity. You need to make time
for solitude, breathing, unwinding and just being. If
you don't, you may end up crying in a dentist's chair
in horrific pain like me – or worse.

If you ignore the messages (read pain) you will
inevitably bottle up what is no longer serving you
and it will come back with a vengeance. It will come
back stronger than you are and eat you alive.

So, let it out and let yourself grow. Don't end up like me, in pain, wondering why it took this much to get me to slow down. You are stronger than you think you are. Just don't let that strength be a fortress of stress.

And, floss.

Change Your Story

- *When was the last time you truly relaxed?*
- *Where are your "stress" levels?*
- *Can you change anything today that could help?*

First stop-the body

"I don't see how a world that makes such wonderful things could be bad." - Ariel, The Little Mermaid

Erasing the self-sabotage years.

The chronic pain really did a number on me, as you can already tell. I wasn't going to heal overnight and I knew I couldn't keep up with my lifestyle any longer. Well, I could, but my body couldn't.

I was led to a nutritionist that could help me fix my body, but I had to put in the work, detox out the crap that was holding me back and heal everything I had damaged. It was going to be a forklift of a job.

I enlisted help because, on this health journey, you can't do it alone.

I had a team of two holistic doctors working with me, daily. I had a Chiropractor, Dr. Valov Vasco, and a Nutritionist, Mike Delafave, on my side. They had a two-part program where they helped you learn how to eat, what supplements to take, and how to turn your mindset toward healing.

And, so I dove in.

Turns out I wasn't eating enough food! Or any of the right foods. I was already gluten-free, and dairy-free which were the next steps — at least I was doing something right! I was eating all the wrong things for

31

my thyroid, however, and I had to change quite a bit around. Right off the bat, I had to stop (or slow down) the drinking.

Here's what I learned (and I thought I was healthy):

- Test, test, test. Food sensitivity testing can be a great start.
- We don't eat enough protein - it has to be at every meal, and quite a bit more than you think.
- I wasn't drinking the right things - ginger ale and booze. Now, I drink organic juices, teas, and water.
- Dipping sauces of any kind are out. Sorry, *Chick-fil-A* sauce.
- Anything out of the pantry (except for a few nuts and chips) is basically out.
- Smoothies can be a powerful tool to get all your supplements in one shot.
- My body was craving collagen, and so is yours, probably.
- Vitamin D is a healer.
- Fruits and vegetables are snacks. Big meals are better though.
- Tracking your food really helps (wow, what an eye-opener).
- You can only change one thing at a time when it comes to diet or supplements (and give yourself three days to figure it out).
- And, be patient, healing takes longer than you think.

I was off! I embarked on a stubborn, uphill journey of ridding my body of sugar-filled drinks, bad oils, and toxic sauces. I transformed my days into meals

instead of grazing snacks. I supercharged my
mornings with smoothies and sunshine. I accelerated
my days with good fats and proteins. I relaxed my
nights with supplements and meditation.

What a DIFFERENCE.

All of my little pains started to subside. My
irritations were lowered, my sleep was better, and
my digestion started to clear. My mood was up. It
was like magic. The power of the body still amazes
me.

Here's what I healed:

- Thyroid levels (T3, T4, TSH) balanced
- Lower TPO antibodies
- Chronic inflammation from 90% to 20%
- Ligament pain from 90% to 10%
- Mood increased by 300%
- Sleep levels increase by 70%
- Anxiety down to 0%
- Reduce thyroid nodule from 11 TIRADS score to 5 (no longer high-risk)
- IBS down to 0% (and a year's worth of inflamed bowels gone)
- Self-awareness, confidence, and empowerment increased by roughly 50%
- Brain function increased by roughly 50%

And, as a result of this my relationships, finances and
overall days are just, better. As the days go on, I am
curing more and more. My eyes are better, my skin is
better, my hair is better…it just keeps going.

**Health truly is wealth, you just have to figure out
how to eat!**

The one piece of advice I will give is to listen to your
body and trust it. At the beginning of this journey, I
did not trust my body and it took me doubly long to
heal because of it. Your body will tell you if
something isn't right for you - listen to it.

Here's my regimen (as of three years and counting). I
am not recommending this, please seek advice from a
health professional, just sharing for those that have
asked:

- 8:00 AM Smoothie
    - 1 frozen banana
    - 1/2 cup frozen avocado
    - 1 cup frozen strawberries and
      blueberries
    - 6 oz organic Lakeland pineapple juice
    - 1 tsp Extra Virgin Olive Oil (Juicy
      Olive Squeezed brand)
    - 2 scoops BioOptimal collagen/protein
      powder (non-flavored - 20 grams
      protein)
    - 1/2 tsp Ceylon cinnamon
    - Supplements (1 Coral calcium capsule,
      1 B-complex capsule, 1 tsp
      Magnesium Glycinate, 5 drops ADK,
      1/4 Zinc capsule)
    - Blend and enjoy!
    - Add two eggs for extra protein (if you
      tolerate eggs!)
- 11:00 AM
    - Cup of organic juice
    - Cantaloupe or naval orange

- 1:30 PM Lunch
    - Protein, vegetable, and fruit (or sometimes a second smoothie)
    - Lunch supplements (Calcium)
- 3:00 PM
    - Coconut water
- 6:00 PM Dinner
    - Double protein, double veggies
    - Nighttime supplements (Calcium, Magnesium, Valerian, Lemon balm, Skullcap)
    - Peppermint tea

I am not a doctor nor nutritionist, but this regimen works for me. I am at my perfect, healthy weight, and feeling great! I follow a thyroid-mindful diet, mostly meats, fish, veggies, fruit, and oil. I eat good fats and sometimes even eat out at a restaurant - which is just fine to do! If I have a glass of wine once a month - so BE it. **You can't live your life in a bubble.**

If you're just starting out or need a change, start with the body. You have to make some changes, and shed some vices - but once you do — **MAGIC**.

What are you consuming? Or what's consuming you?

Change Your Story

- *How's your diet? Is it time to do a "what do I really eat" audit?*
- *What if you took away one unhealthy habit this week?*

- *And what if you added one healthy thing to your schedule? Track your changes!*

In the throes of pain

"You're not dying you just can't think of anything good to do" - Ferris Bueller, Ferris Bueller's Day Off

Love is moving in.

The following is an excerpt of free association pain journaling when I was in the throes of pain.

Some people have money, some people have fame. I have pain. It's been my ruler, my guiding light, and my enforcer for longer than I can remember.

I never asked for it. In fact, my light would shine brighter than most if I was allowed to be pain-free. Pain has dictated my days and my nights. It has been my shadow telling me where to go, how to feel, and what to do.

I'm not going to complain anymore, I said. I'm only making it worse.

So, then it gets buried deep down and becomes compounded upon itself and becomes…worse. There is no escape. There is no surrender. You can't pray this away, you can't make it stop - trust me I tried for 30 years.

Here's the rub. Pain is the thing that drives me to do something about it. It's what compels me to make *change*. It's what fuels me to be a better me. But how do I get better when it perpetually gets worse? What's the formula for constant, chronic pain that weighs me down until I break?

I say and do all the things. I kept saying, I'm everything that I need to be right now. I'm positive, I'm healthy, I'm in faith, I'm releasing emotions, I'm moving the body and working the mind. None of the tricks I pull out of my magic pain hat are working. Where's my little white rabbit to tell me everything is just a dream?

Listen, I'm not perfect and I know I've put my body through hell. I closed out my soul and shut down the mind-body-soul connection — without even knowing it. But I only did it to escape the pain. I wanted to escape this curse that I called pain for just one day. I would have taken even a few hours.

The truth is, there is no scientific one-shot fix-all method for healing pain. It's hundreds of remedies that you constantly have to mix, blend, spill, and even set on fire to heal. Doubt creeps in every day, every minute and you're batting it down with the biggest hatchet you have - and it just comes back stronger. It's like the body says, oh you don't want pain huh? Here's real pain, sweetie. I'll show you.

And then I'm down. And then I'm up.

What's the point of management if the pain does what it wants when it wants? What's the point of maintenance when one thing I do sets it all off? I put masks on to hide the fact that I'm in pain, but who am I hiding it from? Myself? Nobody cares, Caylin. Tell the world. Nobody will listen and nobody is coming to save you.

It's all on me. It always is.

I'd carried the weight of this pain for too many years and it had become embedded in me. Horrifically stapled to my inner being, implanted in my soul. It was so much a part of me, that it spoke for me sometimes. It told me what to do. I beat it down, I put the pain fire out and it would spark up somewhere else, twice as hot.

How much can a person carry before they break? Sometimes I set it down. Sometimes I gave in and let go and it was temporary relief. Sweet sweet relief. And then, the roaring fire of pain comes back reminding me that I can never escape, it is my path.

What if I didn't choose this path? What if I see the other path and it's right there, it's so close I can feel it, but it's not accessible? How do I let go of this shadow stealthily, like a thief in the night?

I saw the signs, I knew the way, and I had the tools. It just needed to let me go. I just needed to part ways with the only thing that's been there for me for my entire life. She had become comfort, she had become home.

To you pain, I say it's time. It's time for me to go.

Thank you for making me realize what doesn't serve me. Thank you for the times you've made me slow down. Thank you for not completely taking my life away. Thank you for showing me that love wins, every time. I appreciate your lessons, pain. I really do. You've taught me a lot. But I can't be your home anymore. You don't own me, you never did. I allowed you in, I allowed you to tell me what to do. But it's time for love to run the show for a little while.

With every tear, with every ache, and with every gut-wrenching breath, I said goodbye to the pain. There was no room for her here anymore.

Love is moving in.

Change Your Story

- *Have you found your life's work? Is it purpose or pain?*
- *Are you in communication with your emotions? Who runs the show?*
- *Have you thanked your suffering yet? That's a hard one.*

My spine, my tree of life

"Whoever saves one life, saves the world entire." –
Stern, Schindler's List

Where would I be without my chiropractor?

I would be remiss if I didn't start my healing journey
with the most important part - my **spine**.

It doesn't matter whether you "believe" in
chiropractors or not (also it's not like Santa Claus,
how silly), they have been a crucial part of my
healing journey. I literally don't know where I would
be without the many, talented chiropractors in my
life.

Getting adjusted by a chiropractor is not just
maintenance, it's a beautiful relationship with your
body, your community, and your state of harmony.
I'm biased because I started getting adjusted at 10
years old and it was the ONLY thing that gave me
relief at that time. Turns out, I fell off a slide when I
was young and my neck was jacked up for years -
hence the headaches. It took me two years to get my
atlas to finally stay in place. Yup, that's the bone your
head sits on.

As someone who has overcome chronic pain, I can say that a chiropractic adjustment is one of my top recommendations. Your spine is the foundation for everything, and if out of alignment can be detrimental to your health and healing. And, no, I'm not sponsored by any chiropractor (but I'm open!).

A simple adjustment can help just about every ailment — headache, backache, stomach ache — it truly is magic.

However, since I was "loosey-goosey", my adjustments wouldn't hold and sometimes inflamed me more. It was a delicate balancing act of hyper mobility. I was very flexible, too flexible. It was as if my body was missing its internal glue. But that temporary relief from an adjustment was enough for me to get by. For that, I am forever grateful. And, that temporary relief became more permanent relief down the road.

My chiropractors became my family.

I will never forget them — their steady hands, their powerful minds, and their kind hearts. A chiropractor is not just a doctor that helps you, they are a friend, a confidant, and they truly know you like no other. I can't tell you how many revelations I've had on the adjusting table.

- Dr. Chase - thank you for helping me to understand that my neck wasn't going to break when you started my adjustments at 10 years old. Rest in peace.

- Dr. Mashike - thank you for seeing me at 11:30 pm because I took a self-defense class and knocked myself into a migraine.
- Dr. Kelly - you saved my butt at work so many times, I owe you.
- Dr. Gaby - you will always be my second dad, and I respect you like no other.
- Dr. Dave - thanks for all the laughs, you got me through some dark times.
- Dr. Grebe - you are such a lovely light, thank you for listening.
- Dr. Vasco - you are my health angel and I am forever grateful for your care.

I wouldn't be who I am without these people, some of which have passed on. And, to all my chiropractor friends, Dr. Amy, Dr. Sarah, Dr. Pat, and so many more, I love you. I love that you are out there helping to heal the world, one spine at a time. **You are out there fighting the good fight, and I'm here for it.**

Your spine is your tree of life — your roots. I prioritized this for most of my life. I know it's maintenance, but so are your teeth, your hair, your car even. Everything is maintenance. I chose to make my body important, are you?

Change Your Story

- *Do you prioritize the health of your spine? If not, try it out.*
- *Are you open to maintaining weekly or monthly adjustments?*
- *What would happen if you stayed in alignment? Would other things fall into place?*

The Eat, Pray, Love goal

"This is a good sign, having a broken heart. It means we have tried for something." - Elizabeth Gilbert, Eat, Pray, Love

It's so much more than meditating.

For fifteen years, I *attempted* meditation. It was my goal to have the *Eat, Pray, Love* moment. You know, the book by Elizabeth Gilbert where the woman tracks across the world to find herself?

I wanted to rise spiritually during meditation and become one with my spirit. I wanted to transcend my body like Julia Roberts. I wanted to slip into the meditation zone and come out as a different person. **I wanted to release the pain.**

For fifteen long years, I breathed, I sat, I counted, I used all the tools, and I waited for the moment of enlightenment. Nothing came.

I tracked each breath, each moment, going on streaks in these meditation apps — Calm, Headspace, Breathe Ball — I used them all. I went 576 days straight and still… nothing. It was like some cosmic joke that I would never be able to reach this goal of tuning into myself. How hard was it to just sit and breathe? Turns out, it was going to be my biggest feat.

I kept saying, I'm not the girl who sits crosslegged in the forest with a ring of flowers on her head, breathing into the trees. I kept thinking, I can do this any way I wanted - I don't have to follow the rules, I can just lay here. I don't have to use the tools, I can achieve this my way. Ego, much?

In hindsight, I was doing it all wrong.

I was turning to meditation to fix myself, to escape my reality. And, worse yet, I was turning to meditation to say "I did it". All wrong.

One day, I was in extreme pain and I dropped the apps and the expectations, and I just sat. I was overwhelmed, overworked, and overthinking every little thing. I breathed into my belly (I learned I was breathing into my chest for fifteen years, *oops*) and I just let go of all expectations. I allowed myself to simply be with whatever came up. I dropped the judgment of not knowing what I was doing, or of achieving some unattainable goal.

Then, a spark happened.

As I was breathing, I felt a small spark that said, *yes, this is it. You're on your way, keep going.*

As I sat there I realized the ruminations were falling away. The monkey mind was quieting and the light was peeking in. It was a peek into peace. It was finally something that I could say, this is relaxing -

not trying to BE anything I'm not. I wasn't trying to prove that I was a meditation guru or that I was doing it "right". What's the right way, anyway?

My mind calmed to a point of reflection. It was as if I was looking into a mirror in my mind and I saw myself struggling. I watched this determined soul, climbing up the meditation mountain that I had built, and she just kept falling. She slipped and slid down time and time again, and I couldn't help her. And, finally, I watched her slowly get up for the last time. She finally took that step that reached the top, and she gasped for air after years of doubt. She had finally made it.

All it took was full surrender.

At that moment, sitting on my sofa, in my robe at 6:30 in the morning, I broke the meditation cycle in half. I threw out all the things that I was told to do, and I just allowed my intuition (whom I had not trusted for 30 years, mind you) to tell me that it was okay to just do whatever I felt was right.

I didn't have to have a process, a workflow, or a right way to meditate - it just had to be beneficial for what I needed at that moment. And at that moment, I needed to be set free. I was trying so hard to meditate for all the wrong reasons, that it just clicked. What's right for me will find me, I don't have to search for it. I get fixated on things so easily, that I totally missed the entire goal.

The goal of meditation is to set yourself free.

Finally, I was able to just be one with my body (my beautiful, aching body) and be okay with my mind (my terrifying thoughts), and open my heart to my spirit (oh, hello). And, it was a magical moment of connection. I didn't realize how separate they had been for so, so long. It was like they were in different rooms, not speaking to each other all these years.

Meditation opened the doors for my mind, body, and spirit to become one again and say - *everything is okay, Caylin.* You don't have to worry anymore. What's done is done. You can come home now.

No matter where you are on your meditation journey, don't give up. It took me fifteen years to realize that it was inside me all along. There is no right or wrong way, just be one with yourself. Listen to the whispers of your spirit, breathe, and just be okay with whatever comes up.

What comes up is going to heal you and show you the way. Just listen.

Change Your Story

- *Have you tried meditation or do you meditate regularly?*
- *The next time you meditate, ask yourself, what do I need to hear?*
- *Can you make time to meditate daily, if even for five minutes? Journal what comes up.*

The rising sun

"The sun is shining on another day and hope is whispering in my ear." - Judy Davis, My Brilliant Career

Face to the sun; shadows behind me.

For years, mornings were the worst. I was historically known for not being a morning person. Each morning would be filled with pain, regret, and worry for the day ahead. Would it be filled with hip, head, or stomach pain today? Would it be filled with anxiety? Would it be a migraine this time? Or maybe sciatic. Sometimes I would wake up with all of it.

Needless to say, mornings were not my friend.

It wasn't until I was out of the self-sabotage era of my life that I learned that alcohol was fueling a lot of my anguish. It was the core root of most of my problems, unfortunately, and I had to let her go. Which is yucky because I loved drinking, to be honest. I was a great drinker! I was fun, loving and really enjoyed my time whilst on the booze. **Until the next day.**

The days after drinking I realized I woke up and hated my life. No matter if it was good or not, I lived in regret and shame most mornings for having consumed so much, for no reason. It would be a

Tuesday and I'd had way too much because I didn't want to deal with the pain. And, we all know, that it was a vicious cycle of alcohol causing the inflammation, and it would happen over and over again.

Each morning I would rise and do it all over again.

I hated waking up, I wanted to sleep forever. I wanted the sleep to take away the pain. And, when it didn't, I would get angry. And, then I would take it out on those around me. I would snap at them, without knowing why. I'm still working through it, still apologizing for my behavior to this day.

What I was missing was the true art of waking up. I wanted to wake up and feel *good*. I wanted to wake up and not hate what I did yesterday. But I couldn't stop the mental need to want to have fun, to feel good. I would say, okay, I'm not drinking today, but then 5:00 would hit and the can would crack open. They say nicotine is the most addicting, I beg to differ. The buzz of a drink is by far the most mind-controlling thing on this planet.

But, what does this have to do with the morning sun?

Fast forward to Caylin, not drinking. The mornings came, and I didn't hate my life. I didn't have pain upon rising, I didn't have shame when I got out of bed. I woke up, put my feet on the ground, and said my gratitude. I got up and stretched, put my robe on, and padded into my little room to do my meditation and some red light therapy. I breathed, did some yoga, and tuned into my spirit. I thanked God for the day and put my shoes on. I grabbed the leash, let the dog out, and hit the pavement.

And the first thing that hit my face was the rising sun. Bursting and blaring with light - just right in my face saying GOOD MORNING, whether I liked it or not. The sun didn't care about what we did yesterday or the day before. The sun didn't care about your pain, it was up there just healing the world. **It burned bright each morning, waiting for me to burn bright myself.**

I started to look forward to the patches of light on the ground where the sun hit. I longed for the warmth on my skin and I'd take the path where the sun shone most. I felt the joy that hit me (and my dog) as we walked on and on in the sunlight. Why was something so small as the light on my face, so cleansing? Because darkness can't live in the light.

Turns out, sunrise in your bare eyes in the morning is scientifically healing. I didn't even know.

If we can get at least three minutes of sunlight in our bare eyes in the morning, magical things happen to our bodies. And, a lot of magical things were needed to help my body. I started to notice that I slept better. I noticed my gut was balancing. My mood was lifting. My body was less achy. I wasn't as cranky about things I didn't want to do. I was able to smile in the mornings. WHAT? Smile? In the mornings? Who was this girl?

The truth is, I just needed something to motivate me.

I became *addicted*. Instead of being addicted to the booze, I became addicted to the sun. What was even happening? On days I didn't have to walk the dog, I still walked in the sun. I found time to sit outside (even in the winter) so the sun hit my face first thing in the morning. I closed my eyes to the light and just let it do its thing. And, I will never go back to the darkness.

The sun has power. You have power. Put them together.

Change Your Story

- *What is your morning routine like? Do you wake up with pain or purpose?*
- *Can you change your story to enjoy your mornings?*
- *What would happen if you got sun on your face each morning? Journal it out.*

Speaking your truth

"Carpe Diem boys. Seize the Day. Make your lives extraordinary!" - John Keating, Dead Poets Society

Authenticity heals your thyroid.

Throughout my healing journey, I learned a lot of my problems were stemming from my thyroid. I'm not sure if you're familiar with the symbolism of the thyroid - the connection to your throat chakra and speaking your truth - but I was not. In fact, I would hear horror stories of people with thyroid issues and feel grateful I didn't have to deal with that.

Until one day I did.

The day I heard the news that I had a 2.7-millimeter thyroid nodule that was very high-risk of cancer, calcified on my thyroid — fear took over. I didn't know it then but fear would be my guide for the next few years as I navigated thyroid wellness. How had the doctors missed this? For years, this mass was growing on my neck, and was so rooted in, it was calcified into place. How had I missed this? It had made itself at home and was wreaking havoc on my thyroid and immune system. Was I that deaf to my own body?

The doctor told me to come back when my hair fell out.

I cried for days. I learned that testing your Thyroid Peroxidase (TPO) antibodies is not routine lab work. Which is why they missed it years ago. Doctors may test your TSH, T3, or T4 to see if your thyroid is functioning normally. This could be all well and good for some, but their antibodies (an autoimmune response that attacks healthy thyroid cells) could be out of control. For your reference, your thyroid antibodies should range from 0-60 (maximum, and I've seen tests that say under 35). Over the course of a decade, my antibodies would fluctuate drastically.

Here's my TPO lineup:

- 2019: 237, 276
- 2021: 491, 648
- 2022: 5,827, 609, 3,770, 879
- 2023: 1114, 1038

And the fight is not over. It will be lifelong maintenance, but it's currently manageable.

Keep in mind the nodule was just sitting there and the TSH and T3/T4 levels were fine. When you get a lab test back and your antibodies are in the 5K range, you let fear win. You crumble to the ground and say, why me? You figure you have cancer, you are dying and this is it. Fold in the towel, you're donezo. And I did.

And then I learned about the **throat chakra.**

Our throat chakra is an energy point in the body that is involved with speaking our truth. How many years had gone by where I have been stifling my voice? How many conversations had I put a mask on to be what people wanted me to be? How many times had I been told, you're too loud, Caylin? It was all connected to the thyroid. I learned all these things that were connected to the thyroid. Even chanting came up as way to heal it. Sound, frequencies, and humming, were all ways to help open your throat chakra. Some worked, some didn't. (To be honest, chanting always felt kind of weird to me.) But I could hum!

Slowly and steadily, I regulated my diet. I gave way to my vices. I slept a little better, I opened my heart to forgiveness. But I still wasn't speaking my truth. **I still wasn't being my authentic self because I was living in fear. Of everything.**

Then I was invited by my nutritionist (God love him) to start a podcast about my healing journey. In my mind, I thought, I'm not healed, how am I going to help heal others? There were days I couldn't even show up for myself, how was I possibly going to be a light for others? But I said yes because it sounded like a fun thing to do with my best friend, Chrissy Rice.

And so, the *Heal Your Life With Us* podcast was born.

It became my reason for showing up. It became a platform for me to speak my truth. Episode after episode, I unleashed the throat chakra fire and just talked it out. I mean, we really talked it out. There

were times I would get off and think, what just
happened? I didn't even know I felt that way!

Being vulnerable was healing me.

I was sharing my deepest, darkest secrets with the
world (even though few were listening then) and I
couldn't stop. My throat chakra was waking up to
this and *loving* it. The actual healing had begun, and
it was with the power of my voice - the one thing I
was told to lock up - that would finally set me free.

I realized I was SO focused on healing, that I wasn't
allowing healing to take place. I was also telling my
brain and body that there was something wrong with
me by applying all these labels. Autoimmune,
thyroid disease, chronic ligament disorder, IBS — my
body was just following suit. It was saying, you gave
me this title so I will fulfill my duty and live up to it
because you say we are "not normal". I had to
change my story.

In talking through my healing, I was also seeing
where I was in my own way. I was also seeing how
my trauma was coming up through my thyroid. Why
was I dead set on people-pleasing? Why was I fixated
on being perfect when no one else is? Why did I care
so much about this or that? My values were all
screwed up, and self-love and connection weren't
anywhere on my list. All I wanted was this thyroid
nodule gone and it wasn't going anywhere until it
taught me a lesson.

And that lesson was, nobody puts Caylin in the
corner.

Literally, through the art of free speech, I was finally able to see what true healing is. And it's not blueberries or magnesium. Yes, those are the foundational blocks to a healthy life. But your mind has to be open to the fact that you are the cause of your own suffering. **What labels you put on yourself ARE the reason for the pain.**

You need to freely say who the eff you are, and not care what people think of it. You can't let fear win, and you certainly can't give up. You can't give your heart away, and expect people to love you the way you love them — you have to just let it all be what it is.

What's left is me, talking into a virtual microphone, letting the world know that they can heal, too.

And, here we are, with hundreds of thousands of views on YouTube, people listening all over the world (to us!?) and so many lives touched. And we have so much more to say.

All because my voice needed to be heard. Our motto is, if we can help one person, that's enough. Right now, that person is you, reader.

Change Your Story

- *Are you speaking your truth?*
- *Even if you don't have symptoms, check your thyroid antibodies — testing can save lives.*
- *Are you open to saying how you really feel and doing the deep work to be your authentic self? Journal it out.*

Signs are everywhere

*"Roads? Where we're going, we don't need roads." -
Dr. Emmett Brown, Back To The Future*

Why couldn't I see them before?

When you live in pain, nothing is joyful. When you're stressed, unhealthy, and out of balance, everything is a chore. There is nothing that lights you up, you simply wait for the next shoe to drop. Does this feel familiar to you? Get up, grind, go to bed.

It wasn't living.

And then COVID hit and the world sucked even more. I didn't want to go outside, I didn't want to interact with the public, and I didn't want to do anything but burrow in. I wanted to hunker down until the world was healed.

I was closed. I was closed off from healing, from experiencing joy, and from living life, to be honest. I believe people call this depression. I don't know, I just was in it deep. I suppose the pain took over.

It wasn't until my Dad died that I realized I was missing all the signs. Instead of going out into the world with a chip on my shoulder, I needed to open my eyes to synchronicities. **I really needed to open my heart to the magic of the world.**

This isn't a mystical, woo-woo moment. You don't
need to stop reading. Hear me out.

My soul sister and wonderful light, Chrissy Rice
gifted me the book, Signs by Laura Lynn Jackson,
and a shift happened in my life. I was grieving big
time. I lost my Dad, my job, and my best friend since
Kindergarten in the span of one month. I was down
and out, alone with my pain, and lost. Completely
lost. You might say, this was my rock bottom. I saw
no way out of my pain. I saw it as a life sentence.
This was just my life. And now, I missed my Dad,
didn't have my lifelong friend to talk to, and didn't
have a job to keep me busy.

**Turns out, it was God saying, it's time to slow
down, Caylin.**

If I hadn't lost my job, I wouldn't have had time to
grieve my Dad. I wouldn't even be open to the signs
he would send, I wouldn't have even known they
existed.

You may be asking, what do you mean, signs,
Caylin? Well, here they are.

For my entire life, my Dad and I used 123 as I love
you. Three words, three numbers. When he died, it
was like the world exploded with 123s everywhere.
They were coming up in droves. Everywhere I
looked, they were there - on the clock, on license
plates, on my phone, in my feed, in my emails, on
TV, in receipts, on the mail, in the tiniest of ways…
they bombarded my life —with love. I even moved
into a house where the neighbor's address was 123. I

60

mean what are the chances? Dad was trying to tell me - it's going to be okay - **I love you.**

I even tested it. A month after my Dad passed, I asked for something unique, something that wasn't *our* sign. I said, alright Dad, send me a giraffe.

Two days later, I drove down to St. Augustine and was stopped at a red light. To my right was a 10-foot giraffe statue in front of a business park. It even had sunglasses on, right next to a burger joint named *One Twenty Three*. I busted out into laughter and then promptly into tears.

More signs came. There was a red cardinal that came to live in my tree out front after he died. (As you may know, cardinals are known as signs from passed loved ones.) He waited for me to get home from my walks, to squawk and say, I'm here, I'm with you. He also pooped all over my driveway — a way to make me laugh, perhaps?

I would see dragonflies everywhere and they would walk with me, right alongside me. I had always wanted one to land on me my whole life, and they never did. Ever. And, just like that, one did, right on my toe. It could have been Dad saying, I told you to have faith and be patient.

Signs were everywhere.

I would start to see numbers in threes…they would show up, literally everywhere. 111, 222, 333 — they filled my life, wherever I went. I would look up at the clock and it would be 4:44 or 5:55. I would pause a video and it would be 3:33. I would see it at gas stations, grocery stores, billboards - everywhere 888, 999. These numbers would show up, as signs that everything was going to be okay, that I wasn't alone. At least that's what I took from it (we all see different things).

But what this did for me mentally was encourage me to want to be a part of the world again. It made me want to look for the magic out there.

It didn't matter what they meant. I wanted to see joy in the world again and this provided me with it. I wanted to know my Dad was there, with me, somehow. And he was. I wanted to know if I was on the right path, and I was. I wanted to know that there wasn't just pain out there, that there was still love in the world — somewhere. And, there was. I just hadn't opened my eyes.

Because I had the chance to grieve, I was able to open my eyes to what really mattered. Nature, sun, time, **love**.

I distinctly remember the day I received strict instructions from my doctor to get a thyroid biopsy, which often will anger the thyroid and could make it worse. I was getting pressure from all angles actually - everyone was saying it could be cancer - fear had taken over. The morning I found out, I found not one, not two, but three (cue 123) shiny St. Jude charms on the street. On the back it said, "Pray for me". I went home and looked it up. And it meant to "have faith". And, so I did. I prayed and had faith in myself and a higher power.

Another time, I was questioning a decision about thyroid surgery, even further down the diagnosis hole - with the cancer scare, it was all so confusing. As I was pacing, talking on the phone outside about what I should do, I walked right up to a gigantic hawk feather - a message from my angels! I was on the right path, listen to my heart, keep going…the message was clear.

Take what you want from this chapter, but if you're just going through the motions, you may be missing out on the magic. Do you see things that make you stop? It could be a bird, a song, a butterfly, a sign, or a number, but does it make you do a double-take? It could be a sign that a loved one that has passed is trying to tell you they love you. Or it could be a sign you're on the right path. Or it could just be a butterfly, if that's the way you want to live.

I choose to see the magic.

Because at one point I didn't see the magic and it was dark. Now, I choose to live in the light.

Change Your Story

- *Are you closed off to the magic of the world? If so, why?*
- *Are you open to seeing the signs? Try it.*
- *What would happen if you allowed yourself to see signs everywhere? Would it change your perspective on your journey?*

Divine breadcrumbs

"Remember...all I'm offering is the truth. Nothing more." - Morpheus, The Matrix

Follow ~~the white rabbit~~ your intuition.

Remember *The Matrix*? Where Neo follows the white rabbit and it ends up being a tattoo on some girl in a club which is where he meets Trinity? Neo didn't doubt the message to follow the white rabbit, he just did it. That's truly following your intuition, Neo!

But was it intuition? Or was it Divine breadcrumbs?

It took me til I was 40 years old to figure out my intuition. What? You mean I have an internal navigation system that I can just *trust*? Nah. My body betrayed me, why should I trust my mind? Ah, because it's not my mind talking. It's my soul.

I learned that we are the director of our mental movie, even if we aren't the originator. We still have free will, however. I was mistaking free will for free everything. I wasn't listening to the voices in my head because I didn't trust them. Turns out, you have to turn on that power by connecting with yourself. It will lay dormant until you open the door to your intuition and stop doubting yourself.

I found this out in *Light is the New Black* by Rebecca Campbell. It literally hit me over the head that I wasn't listening. I kept pulling the "deconstructing doubt" healing card and I wondered, why? What am I doubting? Oh, only everything. I wasn't only doubting myself, I was doubting everyone else too. **Trust is a big thing with intuition, it turns out.**

Throughout this book you'll learn how I tapped into my intuition. It's not just one thing that opens the door, it's many. It's getting your body back to health, it's trusting in yourself again, it's regulating your nervous system, it's forgiving your past, it's tuning into the Divine, it's understanding your thresholds, it's setting boundaries, it's taking the time to breathe…it's a lot. But it's all worth it.

As you've just read, there are signs and synchronicities everywhere conspiring to help you. If you don't let your ego or brain get in the way, you can live your life by following your intuition, and of course Divine breadcrumbs.

What are Divine breadcrumbs? Exactly what you think they are! They are the little breadcrumbs (cue the old fables and tales) that will lead you to exactly what you need (or don't need) provided by a higher source — God.

The trick is that you have to be truly tuned in to your intuition to actually see or feel these breadcrumbs. If you're in the dark night of the soul, you may not see the signs. If you're energy is blocked, you definitely can't see them. So, by getting to health, setting your mind straight, and getting your ego out of the way, you are allowing the Divine to show you the way.

Here's an example of a Divine breadcrumb trail.

You are searching for a new career but you aren't sure of how to do it or when to do it or even if you should do it. It's been "itching" at you for a while that you are undervalued and your soul is not shining in this skill set. Your mind is constantly wondering about what you'd rather be doing and how you want to find joy in what you do.

The next day you read a post about finding your purpose, perhaps it's an article leading to a podcast, leading to a new guru you might follow - talking all about how you should follow your gut and **go with what feels right to your soul.**

The first breadcrumb has been picked up.

The following day, you receive an email from a friend wanting to start a new project that is creative, fun, and right up your alley. Your eyes light up with delight as you start to brainstorm the project and create new ideas about it. Your soul is awakening to like this idea, and you have a spark of joy.

The second breadcrumb has been picked up.

The next week you get a call from your boss that your deadlines have been extended and you haven't taken your PTO so you should take the rest of the week off. The Divine has then opened up your schedule to allow you to focus on this creative project without guilt. It is definitely the breadcrumb leading you on the right path.

The third breadcrumb has been picked up.

And, finally, you create with reckless abandon - the time slips by, and you are motivated, happy, and highly involved with this creative project! Laughing and crafting and being freely, authentically you, because you chose to pick up those breadcrumbs and listen to your intuition. **It's what's right and meant for YOU.**

And there, is the Divine breadcrumbs trail that always leads to a soulful life. If you can just listen to the whispers, the tiny messages from your soul — they have big plans for you.

Follow the breadcrumbs — or the white rabbit — whatever it is, just follow it. Trust it. **It's your soul calling.**

Change Your Story

- *Has your soul been whispering to you? Are you listening?*
- *If you looked back, have you missed any Divine breadcrumbs that could have led you down a different path?*
- *Are you open to looking out for the synchronicities and signs for your future?*

Retreating into self

"So you can go off and rule the universe from beyond the grave or check into a psycho ward, whatever comes first." - Jack Burton, Big Trouble in Little China

What if I liked my mind?

The following is an excerpt from a journal entry after a visualization meditation.

The day is not half over and I can feel the energy weighing me down. I can feel the fear of pain creep into the corners of my eyes. The dark is seeping in.

Instead of giving in to it, I fall back like a military team in a trench. Lay low and listen.

What does the rising tide tell me? **Retreat for a moment into self.**

It's time for centering, grounding and stepping outside of the body. It's time to project away from this world and into another.

The breath leads the way. Slow and steady, the belly fills with oxygen, spreading calmness throughout my core. The breath builds up and falls back, like tides on a shore, the slower it goes the farther I fall.

I release the throat and jaw - *how long has it been clenched?* My mouth slips open slightly, finally releasing.

I am not my tension.

The space inside my mind grows as the oxygen takes over. No more rumbling now.

I am not my thoughts.

The visions begin then. Lights dance across my closed eyelids back and forth like ink blots in a rainstorm. Purples and blues shine bright and go dim, always moving and growing. Thoughts are trying to come forth, pushing past the breath but every exhale declines it.

I am not my pain.

The inhales have a life of their own now, they've taken on the circadian rhythms of time and flow naturally, channeling in new messages.

A new vision booms into view. A silhouette of a lady forms in my spatial vision, glowing with a light blue circle around her head and suddenly that becomes my silhouette and I'm looking up at the moon. Its crescent shape wanes blue light down on me sending moonlight to my upturned face. My hair flows down my back and my face is lit with powerful moonbeams. The energy from the moon rains down deeper and deeper onto me until it stops, suddenly. And all shapes fade into a vast white light.

I am not my stress.

The exhales have a life of their own now. They have driven out any doubts and returned fire to any fears. Allowing new messages to come in.

The visions are stronger now. Faster. The center of a hibiscus flower forms front and center and then hundreds more sprout up behind them, signaling growth and rebirth, life in all forms. It's my favorite flower reminding me to remember the beauty. **Go to the beautiful things, they will bring you joy.**

I am not my past.

And then darkness crashes into my vision for a split second only to be followed by hues of green and blue. Growing orbs on the sides of me morphing into energy balls and zooming toward me, filling me with life.

Masculine energy forms on my left side as my arm and leg involuntarily move with heightened senses. I can feel the presence of a spirit guide sending me love and light, and I'm so grateful. Thank you for the message of love.

The breath steadies and the mind is calm, waiting. There is no pain. I am not my body. I've fallen into the white light and feel slumber take over, if only for a moment. The palms of my hands are open to receive and I am completely filled with tenderness.

I am not my schedule.

And now, the divine exhale. The last breath of a trip that you've been on for years. And, it had only been

20 minutes. The coming back from a journey within.
It's bittersweet as you disengage from the lights, and
center yourself back to the body that holds you
together.

You're you, but you're different. You're new.

And it's up to you to take that light into the day. Can
you carry that torch?

Change Your Story

- *Are you listening to your body when it needs a break?*
- *How do you get along with your inner thoughts?*
- *What if you travel inside your mind on your lunch break?*

Bad days are your blueprint

"Come out the coast, we'll get together, have a few laughs…" - John McClane, Die Hard

Your mess is your message.

We all wish that every day was a good day. But what about when you're having a bad day and you can't get out of it? What about the days when everything seems to be going "wrong" and you can't turn it around? Those are the days that really matter.

Bad days are answers to questions you didn't know you needed to ask.

When we're high, we're happy, feeling joy, feeling purpose, and feeling worthy. It's beautiful when good things happen. It's magical when things are going our way. We don't have to plan, push or resist — it flows with us and we flow with it. So, how do we get more days like that? By learning from the low days.

Our bad days are our blueprints for healing.

Let's say you wake up feeling good. You start your day right, you do all the things that help you be a better version of yourself. Then you set out into the world and it gets smashed to pieces. Everything goes sideways, things snowball out of control and you're left shaking your head going - *what happened*?

What happened was you thought you were flowing, you thought you were vibing because you were "doing everything right". And, in fact, you needed to let go and surrender to what can happen and what it can teach you. If we set out with high expectations, there is no doubt we may fail a bit. But if we set out with zero expectations and allow things to happen *for* us, not *to* us, we will find it won't go as planned at all. And so…

I invite you to throw your plan out for the day.

What would happen if you let the day run the show? What would happen if you laughed at the low points and took joy in the bad days? If you saw kindness in frustration if you saw peace in traffic jams? What if you found joy in pain? It sounds ridiculous. But that's exactly what we have to do in order to learn. In order to heal.

Our low points, our bad days, are the formulas we need to figure out how to truly surrender. When a "bad" thing happens to you, how do you react? Do you lean into it and then find ten more things that are going wrong? Or do you step back and listen to what it's trying to tell you? I don't know about you, but I lean in hard and get angry. I used to go into full rage mode, thinking, whyyyyyy? I've done everything I could, why would this happen? And therein lies the answer. The why.

The why is the answer.

The why is asking - what is it that you're hiding from? What is that you're running from? What is it that you're ignoring - just to get by? When you find out the why, you find out how to slow down and tune in. But here's the caveat - the why is going to sting a little. The why is going to set you back a few steps because you weren't ready to hear it. The why is going to say - hold up, you need to handle some things first, because you aren't healed quite yet. And, you need to welcome that with open arms.

Eventually, the bad days and the low points will be a simple change in the atmosphere. You'll say, *wow, thank you for helping me to see this — to feel this.* Without it, you wouldn't have overcome it. And without it, you wouldn't be the better version of yourself. It would just be you - pretending to handle your ish, then exploding on the next down turn.

Ask yourself, are you pretending to handle your shadow self, or are you actually handling it? Are you processing or repressing? **Spoiler alert: if it hurts, typically you're handling it.**

Here's a quick way to use your low points as a blueprint. Ask yourself:

- What is the "bad thing" that's happening right now?
- What level of low/bad is it?
- Is it out of my control?
- How am I reacting to it?
- And what (if anything) can I do about it?
- Is this happening as a result of my fear, doubt, or worry?

If not, carry on. It will pass. It's not yours to handle.

If it's affecting you, if it's deeply embedded, sit with it. Step into it and really acknowledge that it's here to create some answers for you - to questions you didn't even know you needed to ask. And when those questions are out there, allow those answers to come with an open heart. Only then, do you truly heal. When we welcome our bad days, that's true healing.

Be grateful for the bad days, they are the path.

Change Your Story

- *How do you handle bad days? Does that need to change?*
- *What if you could use these low points as a blueprint to learn from?*
- *The next bad day you have, I invite you to listen for a lesson.*

Drop the emotional baggage

"The things you own end up owning you." - Tyler Durden, Fight Club

What if I just set this worry down?

It took me 30 years to realize that my emotional and physical pain were connected.

When most people say they're in pain, they talk about physical pain, right? They have a headache, a stomach ache, or a backache. What we don't realize, is that emotional and physical pain are tightly related and in fact, can't exist without each other.

I have always believed that thoughts become things. I knew stress impacted the body. But what I didn't realize was that your mind and emotions are so powerful, that they can create a lifelong chronic illness in the body that would take a lifetime to recover from.

In fact, the power of the mind has healed people all over the world. It's a scientific fact that positive intention has healed illness, cured disease, and brought people back to life, literally. In books like *The Emotion Code, The Healing Code, You the Healer,* and

Becoming Supernatural, there are hundreds of stories of how fear has physically crippled people and belief has brought them back to total health. It's truly remarkable.

So if the power of the body can break you, it can essentially rebuild you as well.

It wasn't until I turned 40 that I realized how powerful my mind really was. I hit a huge wall when I realized I was responsible for my own pain. How could that be possible? For 30+ years I had asked why me? Why had God given me this pain? How could I be responsible for the one thing that was holding me back? And yet, it was the truth.

Let's break down how emotional and physical pain are intertwined and how they impact your health.

Enter the phenomenon called "somatization"- the mind-body connection. Somatization is the reason why people who are diagnosed with depression often experience chronic pain. In fact, neurobiological research shows that physical pain is directly related to emotional stress.

Stomach pain might not be the result of an ulcer but the side effect of an anxiety disorder. Which begs the question, where does this emotional stress come from? Oh, it's deep. Deeper than you think.

Listen, we all need a little stress. It fuels us to keep going. But emotional stress is deep-rooted and complex. It's part of your core being and very hard to untangle. No one really wants to deal with bad experiences or things that weigh down their past. I get it. I didn't either. I pushed it under the rug for decades and it just made it worse.

Here's the takeaway: feel the feels. Process and express. Accept and move on. Don't bury it deep down, let it out. Even if it hurts. And, then, focus on health. Affirm with positive thoughts and meditate, meditate, meditate. **Just breathe.**

Note on feeling the feels. It's okay to be vulnerable and to show your emotional side. It does not make you weak. It does not mean you're a failure. You are plowing through the bad to break into the good. It's admirable, actually.

Let go of the emotional baggage. **See how light your life feels.**

Change Your Story

- *What are you carrying around? Do you have the strength to set it down?*
- *Are your emotions running your life? If so, what's behind them?*
- *Are you connected to your SELF? Mind body soul?*

The art of forgiveness

"My Mama always said you've got to put the past behind you before you can move on." - Forrest Gump, Forrest Gump

Your heart is calling.

When something is off and the balance isn't right, instead of reacting outwardly, I've been turning inward. If there's a question in my heart, I ask. What is my heart telling me that my body is trying to relay? Because pain is a message. The louder the pain the louder the message.

I read a line from Dr. Joe Dispenza's *Becoming Supernatural* and it has stuck with me for a very long time. It said that the "heartbeats are the stitches through the needle of time."

Heal the heart, and the body will follow.

Forgiveness is an integral part of healing, and it is a different journey for all of us. Like a fingerprint, who and how you forgive is totally unique to you. But one thing remains the same. The most important of all is forgiving yourself.

When the pain gets too tough, the heart steps forward, opens the doors, and allows you in. When the heart is open, you may begin the process of healing the wounds of your past. It is a treacherous journey and you'll need help. You'll need armor, a shield, weapons of truth, and really good boots.

As you set out on your journey to forgiveness, you will immediately be faced with a mirror. This mirror is simply a reflection. It is just you. But inside that mirror are all the things that no one can see. That mirror holds **your shadow self.**

In order to face your shadow self, you must first shed your outer layer of inauthenticity. This layer holds what the world sees. It is full of yeses and duties that are not your own. It's time to drop this layer to the ground and say *thank you*. Thank you for showing me what the world sees me to be.

Forgive yourself for what you did when you didn't know any better.

The mirror is getting foggy now, filling up with who you used to be. The reflection in front of you is now changed slightly, like looking through a glass. You see yourself differently for the first time and a small seed of hope is growing in your belly.

The next layer of forgiveness is for your past. You must forgive the past experiences that you have packed away in your self-suitcase and have been carrying all these years. Forgive yourself for how you acted in situations that were not ideal. Forgive yourself for past regressions that you cannot take back.

This is a strong breakthrough and takes hold of the mirror, cracking it right up the center. The reflection before you is now split into two. These two selves both carry truth, but one must go. With a heartfelt goodbye and tears in our eyes, we let her go.

With this weight off of our shoulders, we can turn away from the mirror and face the world. Now that we've set that heavy self-suitcase down, we have made space for new. Now we tighten our straps, tie up our laces and get ready for battle.

The world of forgiveness is vast. There are many paths to take and only you will know the right one. It's important to know that the people we forgive are for our *own* healing and the mending of our hearts so *we* can grow. We are not justifying any wrongdoing or allowing others to hurt us again and again. **We are simply removing the chains of it.**

As you go into battle, you are armed with **love**. Your heart is full, and nothing can break it. When you come face to face with whom you need to forgive, it becomes easy, like cutting through mist. It was all a façade.

Because your true self is shining through now, there is nothing that can own you. Simply move forward with grace and a steadfast pace. The light will always shine in your path if you lead with pure intention.

The battle will be long, and the wounds may be deep, but you walk away a survivor. And over time those wounds heal. Stay the course, keep opening up space. Make room for love. And enter the battlefield with nothing but forgiveness.

Fight until there is nothing left to forgive. It will be worth it.

And, beyond the war zone is a new path. A foreign and crooked path filled with valleys and hills, but it's yours. You do not carry the weight of yesterday and you do not hold the future, so presence guides the way. Your heart is full. You shed your armor. You won't need it anymore. You can set it down.

This is the art of forgiveness.

Change Your Story

- *When was the last time you checked in with your heart? What's it saying?*
- *Have you forgiven your past self for what you did when you didn't know any better?*
- *Are you open to forgiveness in all areas of your life? And if so, are you going to be able to use it as a guiding light for your future?*

Trust is a liar

"A heart can be broken, but it will keep beating just the same." - Ninny Threadgoode, Fried Green Tomatoes

Can we trust, trust?

The following is a journal excerpt from a bad pain day.

Trust lies to us.

When it comes to chronic pain, it's not this and it's not that. It's not ever just *one thing* that's a constant throughout your days. It's all things and nothing at the same time. With that being the case, you can't ever pinpoint what's going on with you, to fix it. And therein lies the problem - you have a healthy fear of the unknown. You can't trust.

Sure, everyone has a little fear. But when you have mystery pains from doing the same thing as the day before, you start to doubt *everything*. You start to think, well, if that can happen, anything can happen. **So, how do I trust my body?**

Trust is a liar and a thief. Trust comes into your life when you're feeling good, sweeps you off your feet, and makes you feel whole, only to break you in half the next day over nothing. Trust builds up and up and up and then one day it vanishes like it was never there.

The advice I always get is to let go. Ok, how?

On my podcast, *Heal Your Life With Us*, I said, "Pain has moved in. She comes on summer vacations with me. She's on my Christmas card list." This is so incredibly sad to me because it's supposed to be the opposite, relief and healing should be moving in and hibernating for the winter. Health should be showing up for holidays. And it led me to think about how I frame my pain. Am I really that attached to it because it's the only thing I know? Is it really the only thing that's been there for me all these years?

If so, that concept needs to be smashed into a million little pieces and burned to bits. It needs to go, NOW. Pain does not get to burrow in and get comfortable, it needs to be kicked out and not welcomed back.

And, so, it comes back to trust.

Trust to me is not about letting go. It's about understanding what you're holding on to. If we're supposed to trust that everything happens for a reason and trust that good things are coming our way, then we aren't letting go. We're holding on for dear life. We are holding on to what we know, what we love, and what we want to happen with white knuckles.

Trust steals little moments by tempting you with joy. Trust says, go ahead, let down your guard, you're totally fine to do what you want. And then when you least expect it, it rips off the trust sheet and you're standing there cold, alone, and in pain wondering why you trusted in the first place.

To this, I say, belief over trust. Belief is way more powerful than trust will ever be. Believing in outcomes has literally healed people, where trust has let them fall. Why do you think they call them trust falls? Because you literally have to fall to trust. Belief can carry you home. Belief can be your guiding light when trust fails.

I believe I can heal. I believe I can beat this pain. I believe that there is a brighter day.

Belief has risen people from a very dark place. Believing you can do something - most likely ends up in you doing it. The moment I turned a corner in my healing journey is when I started to believe.

Screw trust*. Let's *believe* we can do this. Because we can.

–

*Shortly after this, I read the book *Trust Your Vibes* by Sonia Choquette and it completely changed my view on trust. I wasn't trusting in myself, yes, but I also wasn't trusting that this life is out of my hands. I wasn't trusting that there was good out there for me, and I certainly wasn't trusting others. I learned to trust the world first, then was able to trust my body. It took me moving mountains, but I did it.

Change Your Story

- *Do you trust yourself?*

- *Do you believe in yourself?*
- *What would happen if you started to trust that things would work out for you?*

Energy flush

"Movement is never mute. It is a language. It's a series of energetic shapes written in the air like words forming sentences. Like poems. Like prayers." - Madame Blanc, Suspiria

What have you done for your energy lately?

I've mentioned him before, and many of you might know of Dr. Joe Dispenza. He wrote a book called *Becoming Supernatural*, and it's not at all what you think. I almost didn't read it because I wasn't into the title. It's actually not at all what I thought it would be.

Dr. Joe has a pretty amazing tale, miraculously healing himself of broken vertebrae using solely the power of his mind. He fully restored his body in less than 10 weeks and was able to walk and function normally - with his BRAIN. After his recovery, he set out to do extensive research in the field of neurosciences, memory formation, and cellular biology. He dedicated his life to helping others use the power of their minds to bring miraculous transformations in their lives. Now, that's my kind of doctor.

He is now a New York Times best-selling author and has been a featured expert in films *What the bleep do we know, Down the rabbit hole, The people versus the state of illusion*, and *Heal*, the documentary about healing with the power of your mind. And, let me tell you, it's mind-blowing stuff. I recommend all of them.

In the book, *Becoming Supernatural*, Dr. Joe talks about channeling your energy up through your spinal column and into your brain at an accelerated rate. All in the name of healing. He had my attention. I was interested in channeling my energy, as you now know, and understood the power of energy in the body to heal. So, how then, had I not connected the energy to the brain?

Ah, the brain — the computer program of our bodies.

Here are a few quotes by Dr. Joe to get the brain train going:

- *"We perceive reality based on how our brain is wired."*
- *"Your personality creates your personal reality. Your personality is made up of how you act, how you think, and how you feel."*
- *"If your personal reality is creating your personality, you are a victim. But if your personality is creating your personal reality, then you are a creator."*
- *"Process of change requires you becoming conscious of your unconscious self."*

I was totally in. So, I went on YouTube to find his energy flush meditation. It was one of the most intense meditations I have ever done, with a series of calm moments and yelling and all kinds of different music that slowed down and sped up - it was erratic! Definitely not your typical relaxing meditation — but

90

then again, we were reprogramming the brain, and, I was in pain, so it was going to be intense.

Here's what happened.

I sat outside with my feet in the grass, spine straight. I took a few moments to just breathe and center myself. I dropped my consciousness into my body and placed my intention on my energy. As I listened to Dr. Joe in my headphones, he said to start pulling your energy from the base of your spine (your root chakra) all the way up your energy channels to your brain stem and hold it there as long as you can. Seemed simple. Just breathe energy up your spine to your head. I did not expect much.

I was wrong. **A lot happened in and to my body.**

With my mind and my breath, I physically pulled energy up my center channel, feeling it move through my body, slowly. It was like pulling liquid up through a straw and if I didn't concentrate hard enough, I would lose it and have to start all over again, which happened many times.

I breathed and got the hang of it eventually, pulling the energy up to the point where I could feel it in the back of my brain and held it until he stopped yelling at me. Literally. As I was pulling it up, my spine curved (I wasn't even trying to move it, it just did it on its own) assisting the energy up to the brain stem and I could feel tingles and explosions of energy all over my body. When it hit my brain, it was like I was on a huge nitrous oxide hit and my vision went starry, and I almost passed out. *Almost.*

When it reached my brain stem, I couldn't hold it there as long as he instructed and I had to let my breath out in big rasps, I was wheezing and gasping, trying to regain control. I clearly needed to practice this.

But it felt amazing. I went in again.

The next time it was a bit easier, with less dizziness, and more euphoria. I was able to feel the energy move smoother. When it hit the brain stem, I wasn't able to hold it but it was easier to get up there. Again, it was like a high hit me — hard. This must be what heavy drugs feel like.

The pain in my body subsided and my mind felt euphoric. Like I was in a cloud. My mood was lifted and I felt a weight had been set aside, like my brain opened up a door to something. It was insane. When I walked away, I felt…different. Like I had tapped into something. **Perhaps I did become supernatural?**

If I can help my brain be more powerful, I totally will. That led me to the next rabbit hole — **the power of the brain.**

Everything leads to something else on this healing journey.

What have you done for your energy lately?

Change Your Story

- *Have you ever worked on channeling your energy?*

- *What if you took a few minutes each day to do this energy flush meditation? Do you think you would heal, faster?*
- *How can you help your energy-brain connection in small ways?*

Brain magic

"I don't know why my body is so intent on sabotaging my brain when my brain is perfectly capable of sabotaging itself." - Alma Wheatley, The Queen's Gambit

The brain is your magic wand.

In my studies, I came across many different meditation gurus talking about the brain. Specifically, the pineal gland. My interest was peaked and of course, I wanted to find out more.

I wanted to master the pineal gland and all its magical powers. I heard that closing your eyes helps your body to heal so much more, and allows your brain to process better - which makes sense for meditation! So, I dove into the brain.

Here's what I found.

The brain is literally insane. Yep, insane in the membrane. It is filled with so much magic that we don't typically tap into, that my head was spinning. I know, I know, these are all great puns.

I wanted to find out how to use my brain in my healing journey, so I set out to find the experts on the brain. I found Dr. Joe Dispenza, who you know I love, the Brain health doctor, Dr. Abbey Houde, and Dr. Daniel Amen, psychiatrist and New York Times Best-Selling Author.

Every brain specialist had one common theme. We aren't tapping into our full potential. So, I was determined to tap in.

I found out quite a bit about the brain.

I read that it's a myth that humans only use 10% of the brain. We actually use all of it. We're even using more than 10% when we sleep. Dreams are a combination of imagination, psychological, and neurological factors. Our brains are working double time when we're sleeping, truly remarkable.

The human brain will grow three times its size in the first year of life. It continues to grow until you're about 18 years old. It begins to lose memory abilities as well as some cognitive skills by your late twenties. And, it actually gets smaller as we get older. This usually happens sometime after middle age. **This is where we need to be at our healthiest!**

Our brain uses 20% of the oxygen and blood in our body. This is why deep breathing is so important. The human brain contains one hundred billion neurons — information in our brain that runs interference for everything we see, think, or do. These neurons move information at different speeds, the fastest being about 250 mph. That's pretty darn fast!

The brain on pain: I learned headaches are caused by a chemical reaction in our brain combined with the muscles and nerves of our neck and head. The brain can't feel pain. It interprets pain signals sent to it, but it doesn't feel pain. Take phantom limb pain syndrome — when the central nervous system, which includes your brain, continues to feel the pain of a limb that has been amputated. They are just messages from the brain.

About 75% of the brain is made up of water. This means that dehydration, even in small amounts, can have a negative effect on how the brain functions. **Drink water, my friends.**

I couldn't stop learning…

Alcohol affects your brain in ways that include blurred vision, slurred speech, an unsteady walk, and more — sure, we knew this. These usually disappear once you become sober again. However, if you drink often for long periods of time, there is evidence that alcohol can affect your brain *permanently* with long-term effects including memory issues and some reduced cognitive function. *Oof.*

And, here's one that made me smile. Computer or video games may help improve cognitive abilities. However, the type of game, length of game, and our reaction to it, all matter for brain health. Gaming in moderation, at the right brain development level, can be beneficial. Can we say TETRIS?!

And, here are some foods that are good for brain health, if you tolerate them: fatty fish, coffee, dark chocolate, blueberries, turmeric, broccoli, pumpkin seeds, nuts, oranges, eggs, and green tea. I do everything but pumpkin seeds. (Except on Halloween.)

I also read that hearing water has a positive effect on the brain, so I purchased a little fountain for my office. And of course, the soothing powers of the sea have a positive impact on your brain waves and mental state, so if you can get to the beach - go.

The bottom line for the brain? **Good health is key to brain function.**

So, how are you treating your brain these days?

Change Your Story

- *When was the last time you thought about brain health? Can you start today?*
- *Are you open to eating the right foods for your brain?*
- *Can you make brain health a priority in your schedule?*

Let go of hope

"Hope is like the sun. If you only believe it when you see it you'll never make it through the night." - Leia Organa, Star Wars: The Last Jedi

Are we done hoping for things yet?

Pain is like a labyrinth.

It's filled with twists and turns that take you to places you never knew existed. Just when you think you're headed in the right direction, it throws you off course. Paths that looked familiar seem wrong all of a sudden.

In your labyrinth of pain, you'll see corners and pockets of hope. You will start to see your path become lit with bits of hope that creep in. And, just when you're about to give up hope, you reach the other side. There's that word. That word that may have gotten you through your darkest days.

Hope.

What is hope and why is it fleeting? Why is it not the driving force of our reality most days? We *hope* things will happen, and we *hope* we feel better - that's dangerous, isn't it? Hope isn't a feeling, it's a way of life.

Here's the deal with hope.

Hope is defined as wishing for a particular event that one considers possible, to have confidence; trust or to desire and wish. Hope is something you want to happen but never know if it will. That's not the hope I want in my life. I want the hope that is going to guarantee brighter days. I want the hope that gets me through the labyrinth.

The truth is, hope is not a one-and-done concept. Hope can mean many, multifaceted truths about yourself that you were scared to consider before. Hope can be the spark of an idea that blossoms into reality. Hope can build bridges where before there was mud.

Hope can be beautiful, but it must *transform* to become something more.

Don't get lost in hope. Or use it as a crutch. Hope is meant to build, grow and learn from. If you hope for better days, you have a fighting chance. It's only when you're lost in doubt that you will let it swallow you whole. Using hope as a crutch can be addicting because as long as you say you "hope for it to happen" you really are trying…right?

I say, let hope go.

Hope can be particularly powerful in healing because it births belief. If belief is the spark, then hope is the match. Hope can be waiting in the wings for many years and then one day it lights up belief that can't be stopped. **And when you *believe*, you are unstoppable.**

100

Pain will continuously create fear, doubt, and disbelief. It's true it can be a powerful force. If you let pain control you, you can get lost in the comfort of suffering.

It seems insane, but you can actually be comforted by the fact that you're in pain. With recurring pain, it's moved in and burrowed, remember? So now we must dig deep for that hope and transform it into belief — it's always been there. And, it's been waiting for you.

Grab on to the tiniest bit of hope you have inside you - whatever that may be - and transform it into belief. What are you hoping for? The answer to that question will plant a seed deep inside your pain and your love will water it until it's rooted in belief. Nurture that belief daily with love, gratitude, and affirmations. Talk to it. Give it light. And *BOOM*, your belief has become a reality.

While hope is still standing there, hoping.

Let belief in and let it guide you. Follow it all the way through that labyrinth until you lose pain altogether. **Just simply leave it behind.**

And when that hope bursts forth into belief, you will be filled with such joy that you had the ability to conjure it up in the first place. You'll look back and remember when that hope was just a tiny spot in your existence. And realize that it was the one thing that got you out of the pain maze.

Hope is simply the match, belief is the fire. Light it up.

Change Your Story

- *What are you hoping for? Can it be transformed into belief?*
- *Is your belief stronger than your hope?*
- *Do you believe you have the power to heal?*

The Grinch effect

"Saving you, is that what you think I was doing? Wrong-o. I merely noticed that you're improperly packaged, my dear." - The Grinch, How the Grinch Stole Christmas

The suffering *will be* the joy.

One surprise on my healing journey has been this quiet revelation. Helping others heal has helped me heal. What a concept!

Who would have thought that the simple act of helping others would ignite an entirely different part of my healing journey? So, how do you do this if you're constantly in pain?

You'd be surprised how the pain dissipates when you're not thinking about it and focusing on others.

Here's what I found.

The moment you open up and share your journey is the moment that you speak your truth. And, when you speak your truth, you open a side of you that needed to be unlocked. You need to release the pain that is *inside* the pain — the core pain that's compounded inside itself for years. When you express vulnerability and are transparent about your true self, amazing things come up and out of you. Things that were dying to come out. They surface and require immediate release — but only when you're ready.

When you start to share truths, people listen. When you share your pain, they listen closer. When you share the truth about how you got through it, they connect with you. When you offer a way out, they learn from you. So, sharing really is caring. The *Care Bears* were right.

It's time to open up. Wait and see what magic is inside of all that pain.

Going beyond sharing, you can offer tips, tools, and tactics to help others on their journey. Remember, they won't be wanting to know how to do it, just how you did it. It's important not to force people down your path, only plant the seed and let them grow it, if they want.

So, how can you share? Tell your story to friends, write it out in a book, share it in a podcast, create a blog about it — it doesn't matter how you do it, just start. Be prepared to feel terrified about it, it's an uncomfortable feeling, baring your soul. You may have a moment of doubt, but ride it out.

You can help others simply by caring for them and sending them love. Ask questions, be present, and be a light in this chaotic world. Wherever you are, share and be kind. You never know what people are going through. You never know who you're helping and how far you can reach. When Chrissy and I started the *Heal Your Life With Us* podcast, we never realized we would get such an outpouring of feedback and gratitude from all the people we've helped. It is so

heart-warming. And when your heart warms,
healing begins.

**If I can even help ONE person, my heart grows two
sizes.**

It's the Grinch effect.

Change Your Story

- *Have you shared your story with yourself? Have you shared your story with others?*
- *What would happen if you were completely transparent about your darkest times? About your suffering?*
- *Are you allowing yourself to speak your truth?*

The crutches of life

"It's supposed to be hard. If it wasn't hard, everyone would do it. The hard... is what makes it great." - Jimmy Dugan, A League of Their Own

I can lean on this forever, right?

I invite you to look at the crutches in your life. What are you leaning on to get through?

Crutches become habits. Habits are formed to help you get through. Part of getting through is pain management, but if you form *unhealthy* habits, you create a crutch for an unhealthy life.

Throughout my life, I've had many habits — mostly bad, some good. There are many different forms of crutches in life. There are habits, there are people, there are feelings, and, of course, there is ego. When we create crutches, we don't have to "walk". We don't have to put the effort in. We just lean on the crutch, knowing that it will hold us up — keep us from falling.

And so, these crutches become part of us.

The hard thing about having a crutch is that when you don't need it anymore, you're reprogramming your body to move on its own and it doesn't want to. Sometimes the crutches are there and you don't even see them. If you don't recognize your crutch it can become a part of you and you can't move forward, independently of it.

Crutches are temporary, however, they aren't meant for permanent use.

Take a look at the crutches in your life. They may be small, holding up places where you feel you are in control, but in reality, all that's happened is that you've built stilts in your mind. Stilts to hold up habits that don't serve you. So, I asked myself, what are the crutches in my life? The answer was a bit shocking.

I was leaning on my friends and family when I was down, I never turned inward. I was leaning on alcohol to numb the pain. I was leaning on doctors to fix me. I was leaning on supplements to cure me. I was leaning on my husband to take on my problems. I was leaning. Hard.

Are you open to understanding what life could be — beyond the crutch?

When you walk on your own without crutches for the first time, it's going to be awkward it's going to be painful but it is all *you*. And then one day you don't even remember the crutch. In fact, you can get rid of the crutch, by simply tossing it out. Because if you leave it in the closet (your mind), you're more likely to pick it up again and use it when you feel weak.

Let's face it. The real name for our crutches is our weaknesses. It's time to be strong and understand where our weaknesses are.

It's time to walk through our weaknesses. What's the worst that could happen?

Change Your Story

- *What crutches do you have in your life?*
- *What would happen if you set those crutches down?*
- *Can you walk on your own two feet, and face your weaknesses head-on?*

Change the narrative

"Change is good." - Rafiki, The Lion King

It's not *my* pain, it's just *the* pain.

Whether you like it or not, words are spells. Your thoughts and how you talk about yourself are the programs of your body. I knew this at an early age but didn't really harness it until my healing journey forced me to.

I recently read in Jose Silva's, *You the Healer* book that we call it *"my"* pain because we own it. And if we take out the possession of this pain, we are changing the narrative.

I had been wanting to change the narrative for years. I had realized how often I spoke about pain, how I phrased it, and where the complaints seeped in. I started to take account of how my mind thought about it and made sure I was using healthy terms instead of chronic ones.

And yet, the narrative crept back in.

If we truly want change, we need to make it happen. It's not going to happen for us, it's something that we initiate and create ourselves. I am the only one who is there for me. **No one is coming to save me.**

So, if the narrative is *my* pain and *my* body hurts and *my* chronic issues, the change is then omitting the word 'my'. Simple. It's only *the* pain, not *my* pain. It's only temporary, not chronic. It's only mild, not severe. And it will pass, just like everything does in life.

Narrative change: This pain is only temporary, and it will pass. Thank you for the message, body. I will use my tools to balance and get back to harmony.

Even in writing this, I have to pause and wonder, how long have I been owning this pain? I joke about how my pain has moved in and built a summer home in my body, but really how long has it run the show?

You control the narrative, not the other way around. If that means that you're focusing on the pain daily, then that's what you need to change. If you're chasing the pain, then that's what you need to change. If you're irritated by the pain, then that's what you need to change. If you're sad about the pain, then that's what you need to change.

There is not just one narrative to change, but many.

How many narratives need to change before we see results? Hundreds maybe, because old habits die hard. We get into a pattern of rumination spirals about *why why why*. But if each day, we commit to ridding ourselves of one negative narrative, it chips away at the pain source. If we build strong walls of change, we can edge pain out.

Take a good hard look at what narratives you're working with and how they may be owning you. When you think and speak about yourself or your pain, disassociate it - it is not a part of you. It's just a message. You are capable of great things. Don't let the pain hold you back. Listen to the message and adjust accordingly. After all, change is the only constant.

And when the narrative changes, so do you.

Change Your Story

- *Have you taken ownership over your narrative?*
- *How do you speak to yourself? Are you kind?*
- *In what ways can you cut any negative language out of your life?*

A rip in the healing fabric

"You want to get out of the hole? First, you're going to have to put down the shovel." - Rick Dicker, Incredibles 2

Must we always fall?

This is an excerpt from journaling a challenging moment of weakness in my healing journey.

How is it possible that you can build and build for months, and then one instance rips it all apart?

I spend every moment dedicated to healing. Healing the trauma, the mind, the body - just pouring all intentions into that healing process - and then *BOOM!* One thing slices right through it like a hot knife.

It takes all the tools, energy, and work to get back to center, back to that healing process. And all you want to do is flip a table. Your mind can't stop from the should-haves, the would-haves, the why-nots....and you're stuck. You're stuck inside the rumination bubble of mistrust. Again.

You think you're strong enough to handle things. You're coming in hot like - I can take it - do your worst. And then you shrink like a coward when one

wrong thing happens - and it's not FAIR. It's not fair
to the healing process. It's not fair to ME.

It's a cycle, right? You get knocked down, then you
ruminate on all the things that you should have done
or said, then you get angry at yourself for even being
knocked down and then you get angry at yourself for
getting angry at yourself. What a cluster of
dysregulation.

How do you get so strong that you don't break?

The answer is, breaking is part of the process. It's the
way of life - you have to go up to come down. It's all
a part of the healing journey. If you just kept going
up up up, you would never know what the bottom
felt like.

I throw everything I know at these times. It's the only
way I know how. I can't live in despair, it's not the
place for me. It's uncomfortable, foreign, and icky
but I build up my shield, wrap my heart up and
trudge on. **It's just me, here, healing, again.**

I was making up stories in my mind, slowly slipping
down the pity party hole and I stopped the thought
train with a screeching halt.

This time I used the Jose Silva mind-control method
to bring me back from the brink of negative spiral
madness. Silva, as I've mentioned, is a
parapsychologist and author of *You the Healer*, a book
about healing with the power of your mind. I highly
recommend reading it.

Here's the method. I took a deep breath in and held it as long as I could. I turned my gaze upward toward my third eye chakra. I said two words that were stronger than my thoughts. *Cancel. Cancel.*

And, I breathed. Then I began to count backward from one hundred with my closed eyes, still looking upward. I breathed and counted. Breathed and counted. When I got down to five, I said, *"When I get to one, I will be calm, my thoughts will be clear and my body will be in perfect health."* I counted and breathed down to one.

I focused on the one thing I could control. **Breath**.

I stayed focused on that phrase and pictured myself happy. And used the words, *cancel, cancel* when my mind wandered.

The mind started to calm. The ruminations slowed. To be honest, it felt good to be in control of something. I breathed until I felt the release of worry and that fear dissipated. I noticed my brain flipped a switch and was now open to gratitude. My body was open to messages of hope. It felt really good. I wanted to stay here forever.

It worked!

I stayed here a while and asked God to send me protection on this matter. I rooted myself in the present and every time I drifted to the past, I counted and canceled.

Sometimes all it takes is a stop-gap.

Just stop everything and sit with it. I didn't *want* to sit with it, but I forced myself to face what was real and what was made up in my head. And, the only thing I could control was my reaction to it. Breathing and counting took me from a place of negativity right to the present moment - where nothing was actually wrong. And, that's where I will live.

Until next time.

Change Your Story

- *How do you react when things don't go your way?*
- *What's your go-to comfort thing that helps? Is it healthy or unhealthy?*
- *When was the last time you sat with your emotions?*

Grief, the anti-hero

"But you know happiness can be found even in the darkest of times, when one only remembers to turn on the light." - Professor Albus Dumbledore, Harry Potter and the Prisoner of Azkaban

Running from it won't do anything.

It's not as if I don't know that grief isn't hard. Of course, it is. It's *grief*.

That doesn't change how the body reacts. The body doesn't understand that it's a mix of joy and sorrow, happy and sad. The body doesn't know that love was there and continues to form around a broken heart. It is simply reacting to you, reacting.

Grief was especially painful for me. Hence the need to bury it deep down. I had to do something.

So, how do you transform grief from the anti-hero to a place of trust? The hard truth is that you don't. You don't transform anything because it rules your senses, your emotions, and your body for a short while. And, you must let it.

You can't argue with grief.

Grief comes and goes as it pleases. It is an uninvited guest in your physical home. The only thing you can do is welcome it in, make it as comfortable as you can and let it leave when it's ready. If you shut the door on grief you'll create a rip in the fabric of your health - a 'dis'ease in the complicated cells of your body. **Don't shut it out, welcome it in and let it run its course.**

You can't negotiate with grief.

Just let it be, without judgment. It's important to allow the feelings to come and go, don't let them get stuck. Stuck energy creates blockages inside the body that create roadblocks inside the mind. Let it flow through you like water, and most of the time it will come out as water - tears. Water is healing, so let it flow.

You can't stop grief.

It's important to be one with it. It is a part of you and it is happening for a reason. There may have been love where there is now loss. That's perfectly fine because where there is pain, there is also joy. You can find bits and pieces of joy in between the hurt and stitch it together for patchwork peace.

You can't force out grief.

Let it come and let it go. It's not going to stay long if you allow it to flow. Remember, grief is temporary and it's not meant to be permanent. It will know when to leave. When your heart has poured out what it needs to release, it will slowly loosen its grip and allow you to breathe. It will know when to present joy in your heart, to replace the sorrow. Keep an eye out for it.

You mustn't stifle grief.

Shout it from the mountaintops if you must, but don't stifle it. Need to scream? Do it. Need to cry? Let it out. Need to write? Definitely do it. Whatever you feel you have to do, stop the schedule and make it happen. Cancel the meetings, reschedule the day, listen, and tune into what is needed because the message is loud and clear with grief. Own it.

You must learn to love grief.

This is a hard one. Seems like an oxymoron, doesn't it? Who loves grief? It's the anti-hero. But it's really not. It's helping you to mend, helping you to recover. It's passing the sands of the past through your physical hourglass so that you can move on. It's helping you to remember that love exists and it was pure and it's still there. It's holding on to you in ways you can't even explain, but it's there. New love will form, new joy will form, give it time.

Lastly, allow yourself to really love what feelings come up, no matter how painful they may be. This too, shall pass.

And one day, it does.

Change Your Story

- *Do you process and express your grief?*
- *Are you healing from when you did not process your grief?*
- *What did you learn when you actually expressed your sorrow and sadness?*

A little ditty about journeying

"We're all pretty bizarre. Some of us are just better at hiding it, that's all." - Claire Standish, The Breakfast Club

Traveling isn't so bad.

Have you ever taken a journey in your mind? I just learned of this concept of journeying and wanted to share my experience. When you go to a far, far away place - you journey.

Technically, it's called psycho-somatic journeying, I believe. It involves traveling within yourself for the purpose of healing. It's a way to conduct an internal conversation and learn vital information about yourself for the purposes of healing. By being in contact with all levels of our consciousness, you will find the answers to all of their questions, good and bad.

During the journey, you go beyond your own awareness. The experience is unique unto itself and may provide insights that are unexpected and revealing. Oftentimes people will describe seeing various lights, and these can be interpreted in different ways. Many people experience a change in body temperature or a shift of movement.

Journeying is in the mind's eye. Try this. Step into your mind for a moment and just imagine you are somewhere else. It's not that hard because you're the creator of your mind. Imagine a beach, a forest, or a place from your childhood. Now, imagine this journey but it's magnified by a thousand times or more. You transcend space and time because you are one with your subconscious. Pretty rad, huh?

When you set out on this journey, you are completely connected to yourself and your spirit.

Here was my journeying experience.

I closed my eyes and took a few deep breaths. I connected to myself — my body, mind, and spirit. I imagined a glass elevator on the ground floor of the earth I stood on, waiting for me. My dog, Sophie, was by my side, looking up at me, ready. I stepped into the glass elevator barefoot with Sophie and the glass door closed behind us. There was only green land around us and a blue sky as I turned and looked out through the glass.

The glass elevator started to rise with white light all around it. On this glass elevator ride, Sophie and I rose up through the atmosphere above the clouds into space. The energy was warm and inviting. We traveled through galaxies to other realms. There was no time, no restrictions, only white light, and good energy. And, my dog.

The elevator stopped on a white swirly star and the door opened. A path lit up when we stepped down on the star's surface. The white light filled my body

up from the soles of my feet as I stepped across this
new realm.

I was surrounded by light as I looked out and saw all
the people I loved there. And, I mean *everybody* was
there — past and present. They were smiling and
waving and sending me love. My heart was filled
with so much joy to see all the people I loved and
lost. Tears streamed down my face as I was filled
with love.

And then, I slowly came back to my body. I wiped
tears away as I felt the pure, unconditional love of
the people there. It felt so real, and I missed them *so*
much!

**When you journey like this, you're leaving the here
and now.** You are the creator of your journey. These
experiences allow you to see beyond your present
moment.

It sounds a bit woo-woo but hey, woo-woo works
sometimes. I encourage you to try it! Create your
own journey to see where you can go. Let me know
how it goes.

Change Your Story

- *Have you ever tried journeying? If so, what did
  you see?*
- *What if you journeyed for your health daily?
  Imagine what messages you might find!*
- *In what ways can you journey to the parts of
  yourself that are dormant?*

Breathing through it all

"Let's just allow ourselves to be whatever it is we are." - Andrew Largeman, Garden State

So, what, I just breathe?

What the heck happened to breath? Breathing is now something that we need to *practice*.

When I first started "breathing" for meditation over 15 years ago, I was taking big gulps of air into my chest and waiting for the healing to begin. I was breathing deeply wondering when the magic would happen. I waited and breathed, breathed and waited. And nothing. Of course, nothing was happening because I wasn't connecting. I wasn't even breathing out of the right energy center. And I was only doing it because someone said it would help. I didn't *believe* in the breath.

Breathing is not actually about breath. It's about connecting. It's about feeling the connection of your breath to your mind. To your soul. To your body parts that are working so hard for you. It's about listening to your intuition and your heart.

We breathe; we listen.

Deep breathing isn't about how long we can hold our breath, or how much we can control. Controlling the breath is just about as easy as controlling the future. The more we let go of control, the more we surrender to what is meant to be. When we control every exhale, we aren't expanding.

I was once told by a beloved friend and trauma-led Breathwork facilitator, Kyle Hart, of Bindu Breath, *"Don't fall in love with the exhale, connect with the expansion of the inhale and let the rest fall away."*

Shortly after I was certified in Anjali Breathwork (controlled, boxed breathing aimed at calming the nervous system) I had a breath work session with Kyle. We breathed deeply for an hour, working on releasing that exhale and all that comes with it. This is what I learned.

In reading the book, *Breathe,* by James Nestor, I learned not to breathe through my mouth. It's a long story of the science of the body, but trust me, breathe through your nose as much as you can at night. See the Heal Your Life With Us podcast episode on "The incredible power of breath" for more information on that one!

Well, in my breath work session I was told to breathe through my mouth for an hour straight! That was tough. It was unconformable, not natural in the least. And, for some reason I wanted to control the out breath so much. I forced myself to sigh out my breath and really try to just let it go naturally. It was shocking how hard it was.

I felt shifts in my body, in my emotions, in my

psyche, the whole time - things were moving and traveling along my energy field. By the end I had gotten through a few rounds of tears and released some things I didn't even know I needed to release.

You see, breathing opens us up to some answers.

Where are we holding on?
Why can't we let go?
What am I hiding?
Who am I, really?

At first, it's holding on to everything we can control for dear life and saying, I got this. Breath encourages you to say, maybe I don't need to hold on anymore and that's *okay*. What if I set this down for a moment and just allowed my breath to be free?

When you breathe in deep connection, you open a side of yourself that is *terrified*. It's been scared to speak up for so long that it's hiding behind huge walls of discomfort. You start out with slow, deep breaths, grounding yourself. Your mind wanders and you bring it back, again and again, until you don't have to. Your body tenses and you release it, again and again, until you don't have to. Your doubt creeps in and you squash it, again and again, until you don't have to. Your belly rises and falls, and you question *everything*.

We breathe in; we breathe out.

And then all of a sudden you're apologizing to your inner child for not being there for her and you're crying. Tears are running down your face and you realize you just want one more day with your Dad.

You're breathing and choking down tears because you realized how much you've held in and held down for so long. So long. You're filled with gratitude for how far you've come and it fills you up with more tears.

And then you just let go. The breath takes it and you finally just... **Let. It. Go.**

It's inside of us at all times. It's trust, it's love, it's connection, it's being. If you've never experienced this moment, it's quite transformational. It's, well... breathtaking.

You're free from the burden of being yourself if only for the moment. You're free from the expectation of handling it all. You're free from being something you're not, something for everyone else. **You're just you, wholly and completely you - one with the breath.** And it's beautiful.

This is why I breathe.

Change Your Story

- *Do you practice breath work? If so, how often?*
- *When you breathe, are you allowing your mind to connect to your soul?*
- *Can you incorporate a steady meditation and breath work practice into your daily schedule?*

Facing fear

"Me? I'm scared of everything. I'm scared of what I saw, I'm scared of what I did, of who I am, and most of all I'm scared of walking out of this room and never feeling the rest of my whole life the way I feel when I'm with you." – Baby Houseman, Dirty Dancing

Fear is the mind-killer.

Have you ever gone your whole life not knowing something about yourself? I have. And it just came to a head this year in my health journey, which is now being referred to as my spiritual awakening.

Fear. That four-letter f-word that we all face. We all know the acronyms associated with it, right?

Forget everything and run.
False evidence appearing real.
Face everything and rise.

Yes, that fear. Fear has been running my life since I was a child and I didn't realize it until I finally started to trust. How did I get to this point? I broke down. Mentally and physically, I broke down to the point of being so tired of playing the pain game. I was trudging uphill for so many years, carrying the weight of my past, the burden of pain, and the fear of tomorrow that I just *broke*. Right in half.

Sound familiar to anyone out there? If you've ever had a breakdown or even a mini wake-up call, you know that it can be both destructive and reconstructive at the same time. But what I learned is that sometimes you have to break down to break through. There is no other way.

What I didn't realize is that I was living in fear every day of my life. I'm not talking about the fear of spiders, sharks, or tornadoes. Sure, we all have logical fears. I am talking about innate fears… fear of eating the wrong foods, fear of saying the wrong thing, fear of someone being upset with me, fear of something infiltrating my peace, fear of losing someone, fear of pain running my life, or even fear of the unknown. I even had a fear of the dark. I'm a grown woman. It mounted up and consumed me whole like a fear sandwich.

And here I am, going about my day, from one fear to the next, pretending everything is fine.

My fear was so strong that it was living inside of me like a virus. It consumed my cells, my organs, and my ligaments. It was moving me like a puppet, through my days and nights, just saying - yes, we are scared of that and that and that. No, you can't be happy, we're too frightened of that. No, you can't be joyous, because we are too scared of what might happen.

It wasn't until I was up at 3:00 AM, not willing to go into the shadows to use the bathroom that I finally said, *alright fear, let's face this, together.*

Why did I have this insane feeling that darkness was the enemy? Without day, we wouldn't have night, where was all of this coming from? I had to do something. This is going to sound extremely silly, but transparency is healing, so here goes.

We'd lived in our home for about a year. And every time I went into the master bathroom I felt a heavy presence behind the door. A shadow. There is a door behind this door that leads to the HVAC system, which I have checked several times in the daylight, no darkness. But the shadows are there at night.

Nights would go by where I had to turn on the light to use the bathroom or I had to run out and push that darkness away because it felt heavy.

One day, I finally said it's time to face this. I grabbed a candle and I went into the bathroom and shut the door. I attempted to turn on the light but my fingers fumbled and the fan turned on instead so I took this as a sign that I needed to face this in the dark.

I sat down on the cold tile floor, my hands a bit shaky. I prayed for a moment, asking God to help me release this fear. Then I slowly lit the candle and said a little prayer. As I was praying, I looked up into the candle-lit corner, and on the molding, underneath the edge where no one could see, was a single etched letter — "C".

Tears formed in my eyes as I realized there was no evil here, it was only in my mind and that "C" was for me - **Caylin**. The fear was only in my heart and I had the ability to release it. I knew then that I wouldn't be scared anymore, there was no bad energy here. There were no demons chasing me in the night. It was only me - fighting against my own fear of the dark.

That one letter led me to other avenues to let other fears go. I worked on speaking my truth, being scared to eat food, and slowly I wasn't scared to do *anything* - because I freed myself of my hidden fears.

Fear no longer runs my life because I forced it into the light.

It may seem silly, but this one act was the catalyst of a fear-releasing waterfall that poured healing into my heart.

And here I am, living a (mostly) fearless life.

Change Your Story

- *What are your fears? Have you faced them?*
- *Are you allowing fear to take the lead in your life? If so, what small ways can you release that?*
- *What would happen if you lived freely on the other side of fear?*

The gratitude torch

"In our darkest moments, when life flashes before us, we find something. Something that keeps us going. Something that pushes us." - Lara Croft, Tomb Raider

Reach for gratitude when there is nothing left.

When things aren't going your way and you're living a life of pain and suffering, how are you possibly able to have a gratitude practice? The truth is, I didn't.

When I was in the dark night of the soul, I was angry. Gratitude had no place in my heart. I didn't have time to be thankful, I was too busy wallowing. I was too busy blaming and raging. It was easier to be in my pity party than to be in gratitude. Had I known what I do now, I would have forced gratitude to the surface. I learned that gratitude is actually a healing modality.

Gratitude is not easy. That's why it's called a practice.

It takes getting used to. You have to remind yourself to be grateful for all that you have. It starts with the big things - I'm grateful I'm alive, I have food, water, and sunshine. Then from there, the gratitude train takes off and you suddenly realize that you have so much to be grateful for it opens your heart center. And when you live in the frequency of love, your whole body vibes with it. It seems cliche, but it really does make a difference. Here's how I slowly worked my way to gratitude.

First, I noticed how often I was complaining. I noticed how often I was speaking poorly of my body and my pain. I took note of how often I was playing the victim. It was a lot. More than I was willing to admit. Then slowly, I replaced each complaint with one thing I was grateful for. It was tough because I didn't want to do it. It was easier to complain, it was dinner conversation. It was a connection point to others in pain - misery loves company, right?

Next, I started to add gratitude every time I was in the car by myself. I turned off the music and I started saying what I was grateful for, out loud, to myself where no one else could hear me. Was I ashamed of doing it? Who knows. It feels silly when you first start, I suppose. For 12-15 minute drives (during traffic, no less) I "spit hot gratitude fire" as you'll find I was quoted in the *Heal Your Life With Us* podcast. I didn't stop until I reached my destination. Often I was filled with so much love that I had tears in my eyes when I arrived.

The truth is, despair cannot live when gratitude is present.

Just like darkness cannot live in the light, when you are thankful - that is all that you are. Even if you have to convince yourself of it. What happened next was truly amazing.

I started to get excited about my gratitude car rides. I would get amped up to get to my gratitude time because it felt *so* good. My heart center was slowly opening, after years and years of it being locked up. My heart was saying, *this feels right, Caylin, keep going.*

And then I craved it. I woke up with it - without even asking! I put one foot down off the bed and just said, *"Thank you"* without even thinking about it. It was like a gratitude virus had spread throughout my whole body. I have chills just writing this (truth bumps, I call them).

Once you start the gratitude train, it doesn't stop.

It becomes so addicting, that it takes the place of feeling sorry for yourself. It takes the place of pain. Suddenly, I didn't have those aches, I didn't have that headache. I was allowing love to literally heal me from the inside out. And the more I practiced, the better I felt.

I got to the point where people asked me how I was and I said, "I am just swimming in gratitude over here" and I meant it! The more gratitude I practiced, the more it infected me and others around me. People started to see my light and wanted some of it. And it warms my heart, even more, to think that I could be passing my gratitude on to others. I would love to light your gratitude torch, so you can pass it on to others, as well

Be grateful today - if even for one thing. And see where the gratitude ride takes you.

Change Your Story

- *Do you practice gratitude? If so, how often?*
- *What if you replaced one negative thought with a grateful one? How would that ripple into your life?*
- *Can you help others be grateful, just for today?*

Being present isn't always the answer

"All we have to decide is what to do with the time that is given to us." - Gandalf, The Lord of the Rings

Are you being present, *all* the time?

One thing I realized is that being present isn't always the answer.

Yes, being present in the moment is a nice thing. But what about how far you've come? Why not look back and rejoice at your growth? And, what about the beauty of the future? Why not take a moment to envision your bright path? It can be a magical thing to sit in your moment and not actually be in that moment — like journeying!

Hear me out.

Eckhardt Tolle, renowned spiritual teacher and author, says that there is no future and there is no past, there is only now. While that may be true, we are both shaped by our past and motivated by our future. Without these two things, our now would not exist. So, doesn't that beg the question - do we really need to be present at all times?

Take the family dinner table conversation for example. You sit down to dinner. What is the first thing you ask? How was your day? Op! There's the past! What is the next thing you say? What are your plans for the weekend? Op! There's the future. So, instead, you sit down and you say…what? Do you like the bite of meatloaf you're eating now? And then what? Do you like the next bite of meatloaf you're eating NOW?

Sometimes, it's okay to reflect on the past, and have hope for the future. Sometimes it's a connection piece.

The true goal is to use the past and the future as motivation - as hope. If you live in the past, that doesn't serve you. But if you use the past as a lesson or a challenge you've overcome, you can become better. If you live in the future, and you're constantly daydreaming of the life you don't currently have, you're not really grounded in reality. But if you're setting one, three, or five-year goals for yourself, you're setting yourself up for success. Rather than being stuck in the present, you're figuring out the action plan to bring you to a better place.

So, yes, be present - when it matters. Your kid's recital, a date with your partner, a walk with your dog - be present. BE in the moment. Feel the feels, smell the smells, see the sights. Truly soak it in. But that doesn't mean that you have to be in the moment when you're doing the dishes. Maybe travel to the future when you're soaping up the dirties. I'm just saying, it's not a black-and-white scenario. There are gray areas here that can both help and hurt you.

The real question is, what are you doing with your present moment? Are you happy, sad, or emotional about it? Let your feelings guide you to where you need to be. Not I *should* be doing this, or I *should* be thinking that. Own what you're seeing, feeling, and doing - in totality. When you feel the feels, just be in it. If you're thinking about the past, and it hurts, maybe stop and ask yourself - what am I getting out of this? And if nothing, what's the lesson there? Is there a hidden message in that pain? Most likely, there is.

And if you're thinking about the future and it's scary, stop and ask yourself, what needs to change to make this brighter? What thought processes need to shift so I can see a brighter path there?

There are lessons in everything, you just have to be open to learning them.

And when you're present, ask yourself how you truly feel. If the feelings are harsh, some things need to change, and most of them reside inside of you. Most of them are fears, doubts, and worries that need to shift. And if you're worried about your to-do list, you need to work on passing that over to the Divine.

Send it to the light.

What will get done, will get done. What you need to do will happen, if it's meant to happen. And what is not meant to happen, won't. It's as simple as that. Trust that there is a time and place for it all - and it never really works out the way you plan in your head - so why plan so much? Have a guideline and don't worry if it doesn't go exactly as you saw it, because it never really does.

Just let it unfold. Easy, right?

Change Your Story

- *Do you practice daily presence?*
- *Do you struggle being present?*
- *Instead of forcing presence, let it find you. Journal it out.*

The ever-elusive joy

"I will not stop living and breathing art just because you need to relax." - Delia Deetz, Beetlejuice

Some things you just need to create yourself.

Why can't joy be easy? Why can't it come to us just as easily as pain?

Joy is the goal we all seek, right? To have a life of joy. It should be easy. It should come out of the box, ready to use. Open and receive. It's joy, here to save the day.

Instead, joy is elusive.

Joy unfolds in tiny moments or slips by going unnoticed. Apparently, these are called "glimmers" - which I love. They are hidden in messages instead of in front of your face. They are the small things that bring you peace, joy, and contentment. It's not what we feel we deserve, it's something we have to work for - make time for.

Regardless of the goal to have joy in our lives, we still have to find it. To live a joyous life filled with worth and value. So, how do we get to the point where joy comes easily?

One way to find joy is to simply stop looking for it.

After all, what happens when we watch a boiling pot? It feels like it takes forever to boil, even though it's the same amount of time if it weren't being watched. It's simply because we're focused on it. Now, I do believe that what you focus on, you attract. However, with things like joy, the more you force it, the more it shies away.

Another way to find joy is to remember what it felt like to have it.

The next time you meditate, or simply just take a moment, close your eyes and remember the last time you felt joy. Pool those memories together to form that image in your mind when you were laughing so hard your face hurt or you were so happy to see someone you love. Really *feel* it. Pull those feelings to the surface and really feel them in your body. What lights up in you?

You can also create your own joy.

Instead of looking for it, just create your own. Sometimes tossing the schedule out the window and going on an adventure brings you pure joy. Sometimes you need to loosen the knot on the tie you're wearing and just relax. That doesn't mean playing hooky and forgetting your responsibilities, but it can mean finding time in your day to splice joy in. Perhaps you can take five minutes to sit with the sun on your face or listen to a song that makes you dance. Maybe it's just laughing at a funny video or sharing a joke with a friend. Joy doesn't need to take hours to bring you peace, it can be in those moments that lift you up - that make your soul sing.

Do a quick joy audit. Do you incorporate joy into your life every day? If not, there are some things that need to change. Joy needs to take a front seat to your worries. Joy needs to become more of a priority for you and in turn for those around you. You have the ability to bring joy to yourself - without looking for it - just by thinking about it. Remember, your thoughts are powerful, so be mindful of what you're thinking.

Say it with me now. Joy, you're welcome into my life, every day.

Now go play.

Change Your Story

- *Do have joy in your life? Are you making it yourself or does it come to you easily?*
- *If you need more joy, how can you actively make it happen?*
- *What would happen if we let joy lead the way?*

My sound healing activation

"Can you hear it? The music? I can hear it everywhere. In the wind, in the air, in the light. It's all around us. All you have to do is open yourself up. All you have to do…is listen." - Evan Taylor, August Rush

Turns out frequencies can heal. Who knew?

I had the fortunate Divine calling to go to a sound healer. During my journey, I was frustrated, and as you know, trying everything I could to heal. But this was calling me like no other, it was really saying, *Caylin, you've got a thyroid issue and the throat chakra loves sound. Give it some sound frequency, girl.*

I started the search, and believe it or not, it was harder to find than you might think. It was through Instagram that I found my sound healer, my activator, and light language angel, Brandee Lynn Jui of Zen Vida Alchemy. I remember seeing her profile and thinking, her light is so strong, she must be able to give me some.

My first session was monumental.

Through the pouring rain, I stomped up old antique
steps to find Brandee in a corner office in deep St.
Augustine. Her room was filled with good energy,
salt lamps, a crystal mat, comfy pillows, and
beautiful sound bowls. I meekly stepped in like a
weakling, a baby deer, peering over the clearing.
And, when I saw her, I instantly knew I was in the
right place.

We got settled, and the bowls were spread. Turns out,
a sound healing session is also an outpouring of
fears, restrained sadness, and well, therapy. After an
hour of talking about things that I hadn't said in
years, we got into the sound bath.

I lay on the crystal mat, **ready for anything.**

Seven beautiful crystal bowls were played around
me and, what seemed like, inside of me. The sound
went through me, reverberating in every cell. I could
feel it in my chest, my throat, my ears. It sounded
like life being reborn. I remember feeling so much
sadness, and resentment for how I treated my body,
as the frequencies flowed through me.

What was only minutes felt like eons, and the tears
flowed easily at the end. In fact, I think Brandee and I
both shed a little tear that day. As we finished she sat
up and looked at me. She said, and I will never forget
it, *"You know you're safe in your body, right?"*

It was the one thing I needed to hear to set me free.

I had not felt safe in my body for decades. I
mistrusted her, I didn't believe a word she said, and I

constantly ignored her. Why wouldn't she be yelling at me?

The bowls resonated with my soul, the talk opened up a fire that I had to put out, and the connection with a soul like Brandee made me believe that there was still goodness in the world. My world.

No one prepared me for the aftermath of this opening session, and that night I was feeling it. I was tired and went to lie down, only to find myself fifteen minutes later, crying profusely and furiously scribbling down letters to my past self, asking for forgiveness, which turned out to be the first three chapters of my first book, *Goldify*.

Yeah, sound healing is just what it sounds like. It heals.

I was able to touch on frequencies inside me that needed healing and opening. I was able to face things that I didn't want to, but finally knew I could. And, I was able to let that light keep shining, as activating my belief system (I am safe) is the gift that keeps on giving.

Since that day, I have trusted more, opened myself up to my shadow self more, and truly believed that my body is capable of healing. **I just needed to hear the words. I am safe.**

I still get sound healing regularly and love every session. Something new happens every time the bowls are played, and it's so special that it's Brandee behind them, she is a light like no other.

Additionally, if you want to get the benefits of sound healing at home you can tune in to any of the frequencies on YouTube or related media sites. Check out Solfeggio frequencies. These frequencies are powerful meditation and chakra-aligning tools. Each one is believed to affect different elements of the energies in your body. The Solfeggio tones only need to be listened to for a few minutes a day for the de-stressing effect to take place.

I recommend these from *Meditative Mind* on YouTube:

- 174hz - helps in pain and stress relief
- 285hz - rapid tissue regeneration and quick healing
- 396hz - letting go guilt, fear and balancing root chakra
- 417hz - wipes out all negative energy
- 528hz - brings positive transformation and builds core strength
- 639hz - frequency of love and all things related to heart
- 741hz - helps in detoxifying the body and promotes self-expression
- 852hz - frequency of third eye chakra, awakens intuition
- 963hz - pineal gland activator and aura cleansing

Tune in.

And, of this beautiful sound healing unfoldment, I have become part of a magical community of lovely human beings. They have been instrumental in the process of healing, spreading love, and truly opening up my soul. **Your spiritual community finds you.**

Forever grateful for the Circle of Light.

Change Your Story

- *Have you tried sound healing? If not, I recommend it!*
- *Can you introduce sound frequencies into your daily routine? Perhaps, hum or sing more as well?*
- *Do you have a spiritual community that supports your healing journey? If not, it will find you when you're ready.*

A healing mindset

"At one time most of my friends could hear the bell, but as years passed it fell silent for all of them. Though I've grown old the bell still rings for me, as it does for all who truly believe." - Hero Boy, The Polar Express

Taking my mind with me along for the ride.

We all know that mindset plays a huge role in our lives. We see it everywhere — have a positive mindset, mindset is everything, build mental fitness… it's the billboard of our life's mission.

But do we actually have a healing mindset? Do we believe we can heal our bodies with the power of our minds? I would say it takes a lot of convincing. For me, it took hundreds of books, umpteen podcasts, and gurus from every walk of life to convince me that my mind was powerful. And even now, I have to combat skepticism daily.

Why do our minds innately go toward the negative? Are we hard-wired for doom and gloom? And if that's the case, how much work is it to reprogram the mind to think positively?

The answer is that we don't have a choice.

We have to work at a positive mindset, we have to work towards a healing mentality. It's the only way - because if we let the negative in, then the darkness wins. And if darkness wins, there is no healing.

Here's what I do to get into a healing mindset, daily.

I wake up with gratitude.
I offer my troubles to God.
I ask my angels for help.
I face my fears.
I lean into my emotions.
I befriend my inner critic.
I make time for stillness.
I breathe through it all.

When I catch myself in a fear spiral, I enlist the Silva method of *"cancel cancel"* and immediately go to the gratitude ground. Either that or I get off technology and sit in the grass for an hour. They both work.

One of the beautiful things about living in a positive mindset is that it's contagious. Your energy field grows and the people around you benefit. You start attracting positivity, you start magnetizing higher vibrations. All of this happens in small ways, and when you need it most, it comes back to you.

One decision can change your life.

If you decide to heal, you're deciding to believe in yourself. And, to have a healing mindset starts with belief. If you can believe, you will go to great lengths to see something through. If you prioritize your healing, your belief runs the show. If you believe that you are worth healing, you will do - be - feel - more.

And when you tune into all of this, your mindset shifts.

You can either let your thoughts destroy you or build you up. It's your choice - you're the one who has to live in your own head. Why not become best friends with it?

Make a commitment to yourself to be kinder, be gentler, or to just be aware of your thought processes. Each time fear nips at you, bite back with gratitude. **Fight the good fight.**

Let the healing begin.

Change Your Story

- *Do you have a healing mindset? If so, what does that include?*
- *How often do you let your thoughts get in the way of what you truly want?*
- *Can you become best friends with your mind?*

Manifesting vs praying

"No matter what anybody tells you, words and ideas can change the world." - John Keating, Dead Poet's Society

It's like holding on while letting go.

For thirty years of my life, I manifested. I was manifesting before people were manifesting, I didn't know I was doing it. I saw one clip of Wayne Dyer, author and motivational speaker, in my 20s and that was all it took. He coined the phrase, *"Change your thoughts, change your life."* I loved everything about it. Rest in peace, Wayne, I am forever grateful for your light.

So, I got to work.

As a fixed-energy person, once I fixate on something, I never stop. You put me on a task and I will ride it out until I can no longer do it. I am consistent - with the good and the bad, that's for sure. **But when I heard that your thoughts carried power, I changed mine.**

So, I dove into the wild, wonderful world of manifesting. I didn't share my private learnings with others, I just secretly started manifesting in my brain all the little things that I wanted. It ranged from little things to big things - parking spots to corporate careers. And I would learn that the things I did sometimes worked and sometimes did not…but always led to something that was meant for me.

That's the weird thing about manifesting. It's not really manifesting if you're heart and soul aren't in it. It's not even manifesting if you're not ready to receive it. So, who says when you're ready to receive? Not you.

And so, I reverse-engineered manifesting to find out if we were supposed to ask for what we wanted, pray for what we wanted or simply surrender it all over to a higher power. This research went on for 15 years. I was determined to find out the psychology of manifesting and how it worked.

Here's what I found.

Manifesting is like source code. It has to be perfect in order to line up with all the factors. If just one thing is out of place, it will not come to fruition. Trust me.

When you're manifesting, several things have to be in place. You need to have fully let go of all probable outcomes, of how to make it happen, and most important of all - it needs to come from a place of love. If you're manifesting out of doubt, you're not ready. You have to surrender the manifestation to a higher power, essentially praying for it - and **just turn it over.**

How do you let go of something that you want to make happen? That is a good question and one I have been working on for years. You have to simply be open to receive. Fully and completely - you need to make sure you're able to make room for it. If your life is cluttered - there is no space for new things. Declutter your mind as well. That takes patience and persistence, so if you're ever wondering why your manifestations aren't happening, it may be due to you not making room in your mind and in your life.

Praying for something requires belief. Both in yourself and a higher power. If you believe that you are here for a reason, and all things are from Divine Source, God, you know that you are not in control. In that belief, you are not controlling your manifestations, and can then turn it over to God.

I've combined both mentalities. I started by clearing my mind and opening space. Whenever I start a new manifestation, I clean out something in my house - as small as one bin of items that no longer serves me. Start with one drawer in your house, removing 1-3 items. And then I sit in stillness and breathe, clearing out old doubts and fears that are holding me back from obtaining newness. Then, I turn it all over to God, simply saying - this is what I am open to receiving, and I trust that I am worthy of receiving it.

Easy as 123.

When I revisit this request in my mind, it comes in the form of prayer. It comes with gratitude for it happening and an honest, open conversation with God. It comes in the form of love, peace, and acceptance - because that's how you truly open up

yourself to receiving. By openly accepting that you
are worthy of greatness, you simply, are.

Open yourself up today by manifesting with prayer.
A radical concept of both holding on and letting go.

Change Your Story

- *Do you manifest or pray? Which do you feel more connected to?*
- *What would happen if you turned over everything to the Divine?*
- *Could you surrender control of your life and trust that you are supported?*

Energy healing fire

*"Sometimes to create, one must first destroy." -
David, Prometheus*

Understanding your energy is not easy.

Raise your hand if you know what energy healing is.
I did not.

Energy healing is *work*. It isn't easy, but it is life-
changing.

Energy healing is a variety of holistic healing
techniques that use the natural mind-body
connection to promote emotional and physical
harmony. By accessing, channeling, balancing, and
manipulating the body's natural energy centers (the
chakras), energy healing supports your overall
health.

—

*The following is an excerpt from a journal after an energy-
healing session.*

Everything hurts. Emotions are burning and the
waterworks are turned on full force. It's raw and real
and extremely difficult. I go down and I go down
hard. Energy is dense.

When the pain subsides and the mind rests, the
energy settles. The pain never leaves the body. It is
redistributed throughout my space tucking into
corners that I didn't know existed.

When pain takes up most of your body, it takes an
energy storm to remove, redistribute and reposition
new pathways. When pain comes in to take up the
space, it devours everything in its path. It takes a fire
to burn this down.

And then energy healing forces its way through the
pain gates. Energy is like surgery for your soul,
leaving you raw, open, and ready to start healing.
New, foreign forces flow through your veins,
pushing calcified toxicity out of its rooted places.
Pain that has been embedded in you is torn and
angry and begrudgingly wants to stay. But the force
of light and energy dig deep into those painful
corners and scrape them until it has been uprooted.
Finally free.

What's left is an open, raw wound, blinking fiercely
in the light. This new raw emotion has not seen the
light of day for many years, and like a newborn is
wailing for comfort. There is no direction, there is no
instruction. There is no clear path.

**You must just be open to receiving and letting love
in.**

New energy forms immediately over that raw
wound, soothing open emotion and reassurance that
you're on the correct path ahead. Pain now is in a
frantic flurry outside your body exposed, showing its

true demonic self, desperately searching for a place to root again.

Painful shards scramble for corners that are already taken, desperately trying to light more fires only to see that their flame is doused with love. And light is the only thing that shines now. Light fills the body with a small spark. And that spark is hope and it's built upon itself layer after layer after layer until it is so strong that it pushes pain out of every resistant pore.

Every fiber of your being is desperately trying to hold onto that pain, that comfort, that home base as it tries to regain control and get back on its throne. But hope, light, and love are now in control. Love moves fast. New life spreads quickly and hope is more powerful than any pain body will ever be.

Healing has taken root. New energy is formed.

And now you are left to decide. Where will you go now that you're free from the pain? Who will you be?

You will be love.

Change Your Story

- *Have you experienced energy healing?*
- *Were you able to clear blockages from your body?*
- *Did you feel like you walked through fire? Journal it out.*

The rise of the Phoenix

"I know what I have to do now, I've got to keep breathing because tomorrow the sun will rise. Who knows what the tide could bring?" – Chuck Noland, Cast Away

Can we skip to the good part?

This is an excerpt from a journal around the feelings that came two days after an energy-healing session.

After the fire goes out, you rise up anew. I call this day the *rise of the Phoenix*.

You are no longer the same person. A new energy has already taken root. You aren't scared, you aren't weak and pain is not in control anymore.

Much like a baby bird, you carefully crawl into this new space with blinking eyes, out into the light. Your body feels like it's been through a tumbler, but it's… stronger. It's a new feeling that you aren't quite sure of. You don't know how to describe it but you feel that everything has shifted. Calcifications of pain that have been rooted for many years have been pulled up and the scars are floating around, waiting for a release.

Hope fills your brain as you set out into the day in your new body. What is this new energy? The brain is still processing new pathways to help you adjust. Pain is still trying to enter, but nobody is letting it in. It's hard to remember those emotions you even felt the day before because newness has taken over.

The rise of the phoenix means one thing. There is no going back. There is no more pity, no more sorrow, and no more pain body. It's time to fully embrace who you've become and that is one thing only. *Power*.

Where there is power, there can be no pain.

Yes, old scars remain. Yes, your muscle fibers hold the tears of yesterday, but your body is now filled with a light that wasn't there before.

New ideas are berating your brain. There is so much to do. Energy in the form of color has sprouted all over your body, inspiring you to do great things. You not only can walk, you can now fly. It's not fake, this is really happening and you are able to become someone you never thought you could - simply by opening your heart to receive.

Love fills your heart and spills over into your day. You want to share love and kindness with everyone you see, for no reason! You see the colors of the trees for the first time, you feel the breeze on your face and it's magical. There is no rush, there is no resistance. **You're here.**

And suddenly the day fills with gratitude. You're so thankful that you're not in pain, you do more, you *are* more. You are moved by small acts of kindness, you're motivated to be a better person. It's part of your path to see, finally, to see it all. And most importantly, you trust. You know there is a better path ahead for you now, you see it clearly - *where has that been the whole time?* **It's always been there, it was just blocked by the pain.**

And as you look back you see pain sitting there, outside your door, waiting patiently.

Change Your Story

- *Have you risen yet? If not, what will it take for you to rise up?*
- *What did you shed that allowed you to step into your power?*
- *What new way will you use your wings?*

Downtime is not a waste of time

"I figure life's a gift, and I don't intend on wasting it." - Jack Dawson, Titanic

Rest isn't what you think it is.

Over the last few years, I've had numerous signs to slow down.

At one point, I was running around as if I was three people in one. I had three jobs and two side hustle campaigns running — and wasn't sleeping. I was drinking every night and even more on the weekends. I would wake up on Sunday and ask myself, is it too early to start drinking?

I was in such hustle mode that I didn't even make time to breathe, let alone slow down.

This is hustle culture. I thought if I can just keep going, I don't have to feel. If I can add one more thing to my plate, I will feel value. But the items on my list just kept adding up. The nights kept going by sleepless.

As you can imagine, my body started to deteriorate, with pain leading the way. I had not slowed down in decades. I had not taken the time to ground my energy in *more than ten years*. I had not even taken a moment to breathe.

The universe doesn't give you a small message when it wants you to slow down. It literally sits you down. The message is so strong that it comes through the only way you will listen – your health.

You go so fast that you can't possibly understand how this could happen to you. But you're not doing anything for yourself. Your health is an indicator of your lifestyle, a mirror, a reflection of who you need to be.

The truth about it is, slowing down, is the only way in which you will truly thrive. It is the to-do list. It is the planner, the calendar, and the schedule.

If you allow stillness to come, you allow insights to come. If you allow time to yourself, you're giving back to your health. If you allow moments of mindfulness in, you're listening, tuning in, connecting.

Slowing down doesn't mean being lazy on the couch. It doesn't mean binging TV. It doesn't mean doom-scrolling your feeds. It means shutting down everything else so you can shut down yourself. It means that you're giving yourself space for *new*. It means that you're allowing yourself to process what you constantly absorb.

All you need to do is listen.

Slowing down, includes five minutes of breathing, five minutes of sitting without your phone, five

minutes of listening to music without movement,
five minutes of walking away — just anything *away
from it all.*

When you slow down, all the things that you've been
fearing, doubting, and wondering come to light.
They come out and are ready to help you see the path
ahead.

Also, vacations can help to rebalance, clear out old
patterns, and bring new ideas to light. Don't be
afraid to get away sometimes - guilt-free. That's the
important part.

So, I ask. Are you slowing down?

Change Your Story

- *Do you incorporate self-care into your daily routine?*
- *How often do you slow down? Do you see the benefits of this?*
- *The next time you slow down, can you connect your mind-body-soul together in harmony?*

The Reiki high

"The best love is the kind that awakens the soul and makes us reach for more, that plants a fire in our hearts and brings peace to our minds, and that's what you've given me." – Noah, The Notebook

It was then I knew it was real, it was all real.

What happened to me is truly something that I have a hard time putting into words. For lack of a better term, a transformation occurred during a Reiki session in the spring of 2023.

As you've read, I've experienced chronic pain for 30 some odd years, including physical, emotional, and mental pain. I've been searching for some missing link, or the answer to my pain for decades, and thought I had been through it all. I went down the route of Western medicine, Eastern medicine, spiritual, and all things healing and they all played a very big role.

Recently on my list was energy healing - and as you read, had been an up and down journey so far for me. As I was learning that everything is energy, I learned that we can manipulate the energy that we possess. I also learned that light workers walk this earth, and carry a divine gift. There are people that have been touched by God that are now helping others to heal. This I know to be true.

A quick note about this - there are false healers out there claiming to be real. You do need to have a keen eye and listen to your intuition on this because they will take your money and leave you with nothing. I've had several experiences where either I was closed to it or they were not the real deal. In this case, however, it was the real deal.

Peg Driscoll of *YoRei Life* came to me through a Divine connection with Chrissy who had taken her Reiki training.

As I sat in a car before the session, I asked God and my spirit guides to be with me, not knowing if they even existed. I prayed for some sort of relief from my pain.

I walked in, and it was just like any other office — chairs, lamps, tables. Peg welcomed me in and began talking a mile a minute about all of these messages from Divine. Being open, I furiously wrote notes, wondering what was happening and trying my best to flow with it — to truly believe.

I had no idea what I was getting into as I lay on that Reiki table, but I snuggled in with the blanket and eye mask, and I opened my palms to receive. The music began, and I could hear Peg shuffling around me, moving energy, as she started her flow. I felt both of her hands at my feet, and within seconds, I felt the touch of another hand on my shoulder. My brain went to Peg - still at my feet - both hands on my feet. How could there be a hand on my shoulder?

My heart started racing. My whole body started tingling, and I almost jumped off the table. Soon came another hand on my head, and a hand on my hand, Peg was always in a different area of my body. She was nowhere near where these hands touched me. All of the horror movies I had witnessed sprang to life in my mind and fear took over for me. I prayed for lightness, holiness, and serenity - I prayed it was God's work. And thank goodness for my breathwork training - it got me through. I breathed like never before.

As my heart rate slowed, the touches kept coming. It seemed like forever as she wooshed and whirled by me - performing psychic surgery. And throughout, there were touches, here and there - in all the places of me that were broken. I went into complete surrender and just said thank you. Thank you for your help, thank you for guiding me here, and thank you for the light you're sharing. **Take my pain.**

And as I got up off the table, I was shaking, raw and open. It felt as if I had just gotten out of surgery for real. Regaining my senses, I was in a fog - wondering what had just happened. Had God and my spirit guides come to save me?

Turns out, they did.

It's been a long time since my Reiki session with Peg. My pain is now practically non-existent. My life force had been restored. My eyes could truly see, my intuition could feel and my body could finally regenerate. My temperatures went up to normal, my body rejected old supplements that were no longer needed, and my stomach aches vanished. I started to flow with my life, instead of against it. **It was unbelievable.**

I refer to this moment as being touched by God and his angels. I have a powerful force behind me and I am not in this alone. Healing is not linear - it is spacial. It is everywhere. If you're open to it.

And to this day, I remain 90% pain-free. Nay, I remain **free**.

Change Your Story

- *Have you ever had Reiki energy healing before? If not, I highly recommend it!*
- *What would happen if you cleared your energy daily, weekly or monthly?*
- *If and when you have an energy healing session, what did you overcome, let go or invite in?*

My psychic readings

"Everything is possible, even the impossible." - Mary Poppins, Mary Poppins Returns

Nothing is ever what you think it is.

Before you judge me, think about expanding your mind to all possibilities. If we have flying planes, shooting stars, and now AI (artificial intelligence), we can listen to a psychic reading.

For years, I avoided all psychic information - because I grew up in the era of Miss Cleo. The scam artists ran rampant out there, delving out misinformation to hungry souls. I dismissed it all as hullabaloo. But, when you're on a spiritual journey, these types of things just find you.

So, there I sat, late one evening, on the phone with Rebecca, the psychic. She came highly recommended as a referral from a trusted source, so I took a breath, opened my mind, and answered the call. She had my photo to meditate on, and we all know she had social media accounts to view because I post my healing journey literally everywhere. However, she said nothing about any of that.

I actually didn't speak for most of the call. I listened as messages about my past, present, and future came pouring in — from God, she said. She told me about my light as a child, those that had passed, and how I am a powerhouse of energy. She said my thyroid was my anchor to the earth and that I am here to tell my journey of healing to help others. All true.

With Divine messages from loved ones that had crossed over, she shared that there is a lot of love and support happening — and most importantly, I am not alone. What a relief - I can finally set down some of these burdens I carry, and trust that God and his angels got my back.

Five pages of scribbled notes later and I found that I was completely enthralled. Tears were flowing down my face, truth bumps were up and down my arms, and I was just completely floored. When you think of a reading, you think you'll hear some logical things, even some scary things, but no, this was all love, all light.

It was just the thing I needed to hear to keep going.

Since then, I've had a few readings and each one has brought me to tears on how accurate it was. It helps me to face things that I have been hiding from or were right in front my face the whole time. I was told to be proud of my story, and that it would be the way that helps heal others. Hence this book.

If you find the true healers of the world and trust me, they are out there, you can go to places that you didn't know you needed to visit. It can open doors for you to see things in a new light, and to understand things about yourself that are hidden — even from you.

And if you can just step outside of skepticism for one moment, **you can allow yourself to believe**. Believe that you are powerful, you're filled with love, you have support, and you are destined for greatness. You can sit back and revel at how far you've come, you can stop the worry and doubt of what is to come and you can just simply trust.

Take a chance on healers. Take what you can out of it; it's not concrete science, it's organic information, just like you and I. Pull the threads into the fabric of your own life, and weave your own future.

Sometimes you just need a little help from your Earth angels.

Change Your Story

- *Have you ever had a reading? If so, what came out of it that changed things for you?*
- *What would happen if you stepped outside of your comfort zone and allowed angels in to help?*
- *Are you open to understanding more than you can see with your naked eye?*

Guided dream state

"Close your eyes and pretend it's all a bad dream. That's how I get by." - Jack Sparrow, The Pirates of the Caribbean: At World's End

Is it possible to influence your dreams? I wanted to find out.

For the past year, I've been writing my dreams down in a 'dream journal'. It's been quite interesting, to say the least.

I read a book called *The Healing Wisdom of Dreams* by Kathleen Webster O'Malley and the tagline was, *'Discover Your True Self through Lucid Dreaming, Journaling, and Visioning'*. I didn't want to master anything, I just wanted to try to interpret my own dreams…well that ended up being a journey in and of itself.

Every night when I laid down to sleep, I used the Dr. Jose Silva method to tap into the Alpha brain. I lay there, eyes closed, breathing deeply for a few minutes. When I feel my heart rate lower, I begin the countdown from 100 down to 0. I counted backwards slowly. Then I stop and say, *"When I reach 0 I will be ready for a full night's rest, where my dreams will have messages needed to further my healing journey"*. And sometimes I would add any health wishes or manifestations to the end, along with my signature closing, *"And so it is"*.

Then I count down to zero and repeat the phrase, *"every day I'm healthier and healthier in every way"*. And in my mind's eye, I picture myself at the beach, happy, carefree, and pain-free. I do this until I feel the slow steady synchronization of mind-body connection. This usually lulls me off to sleep with more deep long breaths.

The dreams come like wildfire.

Often I will have multiple dreams per night, whereas before I could barely remember even one. These dreams are wildly vivid, with colorful details. They are strong with messages, people, and places. They also seem to be more cohesive than before, not as outrageous. They are grounded in situational activities, people telling me specific things, and colors that pop out like crazy.

The trick is to remember them. Here's what I did.

The dream journal entry has to happen within seconds of you waking up, otherwise, it will vanish into the abyss of the mind. So, I roll over and with one eye open, I furiously write all the things I can remember. I've found that they are often 10-15 sentences, sometimes multiple dreams meshed into one entry. The important things I remember come to the surface when I write.

Here are the themes I've found from over a year of journaling my dreams:

- The people present are 9 times out of 10 people I know. I rarely dream of strangers.

- The way colors appear in dreams is by objects - so red hoodie, blue bottle, green hat.
- Conversations don't really happen, but words are spoken in one-sentence increments.
- Children and kids are often a theme - many times I'm teaching them.
- Animals are in 90% of my dreams in some way, shape, or form.
- Water is a prominent theme and it comes in many forms.
- Ladders, hills, and stairs are a big part of my storylines as well.

And those are just some of the themes I'm beginning to remember. As much as my dreams are random and crazy just like yours probably are, they often are interpreted on an emotional level, instead of logical. So, if I'm on a boat, and I can't climb the little ladder to get out, it may have to do with fear and overwhelm - and nothing to do with boats. You feel me?

Most important are the **messages**. I receive bountiful messages from the Divine, spirit guides, and probably myself. I may go into sleep asking a specific question and get my answer that night.

The messages come in all forms. A few times they were literally blown into my ear, shouted at my face, or even said over and over and over again until I got it. I would wake up and say, *OKAY, I GOT IT.*

Also, if you don't remember your dream, you weren't supposed to, so you have to let those go. **And if your dream becomes a nightmare, those are also messages - big ones that you have to face.** Your best bet is to ask a trusted source for their interpretation because they may see things you don't. Be careful with that though - who you ask is important.

A few of our *Heal Your Life With Us* ideas came through in my dreams, those are really special.

The moral of this dreamy story? You can interpret your own dreams, and you can even navigate their content. By tapping into the Alpha brain, you're talking to your subconscious on another level, and **it will listen**.

Ready to master your dreams?

Change Your Story

- *Do you follow your dreams? If so, do they include messages?*
- *What would happen if you were to actively ask God for messages in your dreams?*
- *Do you have the determination to keep a dream journal? If so, imagine the messages…*

Turning it all over

"The world is quieter now. We just have to listen. If we listen, we can hear God's plan." - Anna, I Am Legend

It's so nice to know we have support.

Reading and learning is a slight obsession I've had since I was young. The minute I got my library card, it was on. And so, the self-learning lifestyle began, filled with millions of books, videos, and podcasts - all in the name of healing.

Throughout this book, I share an inexhaustible list of resources that can blow your mind, body, and soul, quite literally. There have been times I'm reading something and it has literally changed my life so drastically that **I will never be the same.**

One of these books was *Outrageous Openness* by Tosha Silver. It was recommended to me at my life-changing Reiki session by Peg Driscoll. She said my spirit guides needed me to read it as well as her other book, *It's Not Your Money*. And, of course, I read them all, including her other one, *Change Me Prayers*.

Each of her books spoke to my soul on such a level that I walked away from them a different person. Tosha has a beautiful way of viewing life, having

185

suffered herself, she found her way through it all to truly live and appreciate the magic of life.

One of the things that really resonated with me is the way she considered manifesting. It wasn't repeating that you deserved it over and over (something I had done for decades), it was more about turning it over to the Divine. By simply turning over your desires to God, you are just relaying the message that you are open. It was almost a relief to learn this. **Manifesting was starting to get exhausting, to be honest.**

If I could just turn over my whole day, my whole life, to God, I could finally take a beat. I could finally say, phew, that's out of my hands but I trust it will unfold exactly as it was meant to be. And so it is.

And so I began to turn it over in small ways. I would be looking for something and I would close my eyes and say, turning this one over to you, God, because I knew it could be frustrating if I didn't find whatever was so important in the moment. I went out into uncharted restaurant territory and turned over clear roads, open parking spots, and good wait staff, oh, and the perfect table with a view. I just threw it all out there and said, **I trust that the Divine has it covered.**

What happens when you finally surrender is quite beautiful. The funny thing was, I thought I was surrendering already but no, being okay with skipping your vitamins is not letting go. You have to truly say, let my soul guide me. And see where it takes you. It is fully surrendering to what may come, without any control. To truly believe that you're not in control is key. What a weight off your shoulders, honestly.

And that small mindset shift was the key to transforming my health.

The amount of balance that happened was surprising. I noticed that without doubts, worry or control, things fell into place quite easily. And when they didn't, there was always a lesson, a detour or a reason for it. My mind started to like it.

And when our minds like something, our bodies tend to follow.

When I wake up now I often say I am turning over the day to God. Thanks for putting it all together, I'm just here for the show. Let's go.

Change Your Story

- *What can you turn over to God?*
- *What would happen if you were to trust in good things happening to you instead of waiting for the other shoe to drop?*
- *Are you capable of surrendering control to the Divine and watching it all happen FOR you?*

Bonfire of love

"Ff - flame - flames. Flames, on the side of my face, breathing, breathless, heaving breaths. Heaving breaths…" - Mrs. White, Clue

Light em' up!

Just one more from Tosha. The term 'bonfire of love' came from her book *Outrageous Openness*, and oh, what a book it is. If you want to see life from a different perspective, read this book. It's not only a wild ride, it's a magical one too.

She tells the story of the time she was trying to let go of something big in her life. A physical object held so much weight that she knew she needed to get rid of it. But it wouldn't be enough to just pitch it, it needed to be *burned*. It needed to be lit on fire, never to return.

And, so she went to the ocean, not yet knowing how she would burn it, perhaps she would just let it float out to sea. Well, the Divine had other plans, and in the middle of nowhere there was a huge bonfire with a few friendly guys (angels?) having a good old time, right on the beach. Fires on the beach were unheard of where she was from, apparently. And, with a brave decision, she approached them and asked if she could borrow their fire for a moment.

And, so it went - into the fire! Her new friends were whooping and hollering for her - and she knew it had truly been released.

I've burned a lot of things on my healing journey.

At first it feels silly, it's not as ritualistic as it seems. You have your bowl with tin foil, your fire starter and it's on your porch, in the middle of the suburbs - it's so not magical or mystical. Then, when you jump into the reason you're burning it in the first place, that all falls away. When the fire gets lit and the flame eats away at what is burning you, it does something to you that you can't quite comprehend.

A release.

Burning through your feelings is a very cathartic way to let things go. The ashes that rise up are a representation of what is leaving — they are just that, ashes in the wind. Dust. Nothingness. And you finally realize it doesn't have a hold over you any longer.

The point of this bonfire of love is that even if you don't know what's best for you, God does. We don't need to control it all, in fact, we need to surrender it all. If we can turn it over to the Divine, we can have complete faith that what is meant for us, or what is already written, is going to happen whether we control it or not. It's not up to us.

The hardest thing in the world is surrender, unfortunately.

It seems so easy! Just hand the keys over and let God drive. So easy, right? Nope. The ego has something to say about that, and so does the mind. The heart tries, but it's not enough. The whole mind body soul trifecta has to surrender completely. And then, only then, can you really heal.

Are you holding onto things that you need to release? Do you need a bonfire of love in your life? If so, light em' up. Life is too short to be hanging on to old beliefs and possessions that are weighing you down.

The main theme throughout her book is to release control, detach, and turn it all over to God. The real question is, can you actually do that? Is it possible that we can live a life of true surrender? If so, I've been doing it all wrong. For many years.

If this is the case, then what do I need to surrender from?

Bad days must simply be ill communication with the Divine, and yourself. But, the good news is you don't have to carry the burden of control.

So let's see what happens when Divine takes the reins.

She says, here's the real test. Can you grab a bag, hop into the car and just drive to any destination without a plan? Honestly, I don't know if I could do it, but I'm willing to try.

What needs releasing in your life? Is there a physical object or possession that needs to be burned? Are you holding on to old energy? Maybe it's time to light it up.

Burn, baby, burn.

Change Your Story

- *Have you been holding on to something you need to let go of?*
- *What would happen if you were to release it?*
- *Are you open to writing your past a letter and burning it? Try it out.*

The essential energy portal

"Some places are like people; some shine and some don't." - Dick Hallorann, The Shining

A Schumann resonance response.

Have you ever found yourself in a situation where you're asking yourself, how did I get here? This was one of those instances as I looked around me at the Essential Energy Spa, in St. Augustine, Florida, as it dawned on me that this was not a spa in the traditional sense.

The Essential Energy Spa was a portal. Divine breadcrumbs had led to an energy vortex portal on a Wednesday night at 6:30 pm for some reason.

Who doesn't want to see a portal?

I walk in, slip off my flip flops, store my purse, and am led around this energy spa — vortex portal of healing powers — and I see zen wallpaper, bamboo, waterfalls, and pillows, and then I see it. Four-corner pillars of televisions stacked on top of each other, like technology flapjacks. Six screens were stacked in a black shelving unit in four corners of this semi-circular room. They were all on and omitted very colorful waves of flowing text, almost like sonogram images. The colors were mesmerizing.

With an open mind, I entered and sat in the comfy chair, and looked around. I wasn't sure if I should stare directly at the screens, I mean, we've been taught to reduce screen time, right? The lights were dim, the energy was calm and the people filed in around me for an introductory talk about the spa. I followed suit.

After listening to the sound bowls calming energy, the lights went on and the Schumann show began. Apparently, the essential energy spa was not the only one in existence and there were in fact, several around the country - all with healing powers. The wonderfully spirited woman shared a very scientific presentation and if you asked me to explain it, I simply could not. But here's what I got out of it.

By using the frequencies of the Earth — it's heartbeat, if you will — and channeling it through the televisions, we are able to form a healing portal of energy (marked by an *x* on the ground with blue tape). It had to do with the entire Universe, galaxies of energy, and I must say, it did make sense, on a multidimensional level.

I sat there, breathing, absorbing, and comprehending. Was this meant to be a healing portal for *me*? Was I led here to accelerate my healing? Possible.

And, so, with an open heart, I accepted all of it. And, in the end, there were instructions to take a detox bath to rid your body of any negative ions that may be coming up, post-session. I followed the rules.

And to my astonishment, I felt the toxicity leaving my body the next morning! The healing acceleration had purged my body the next day and I *felt* it. It felt like little dark energies leaving in small ways - nausea, vertigo, irritation. And then, it stopped. It was there, then it was gone. And, I felt lighter.

The essential energy spa had been a scientific portal of healing energy, like an all natural cancer curing center. One cool thing I learned about the television towers — they were omitting colors of the chakras and the text was Sanskrit! I marveled at how it's all connected.

And, now it was at my fingertips!

By being open to new things (even if they are portals) you can allow new ways to heal. Allow God to lead you to these new things, with an open heart. You never know unless you try it for yourself, right?

If you have an essential energy spa (search Schumann resonance frequency spa) near you, try it out! Be adventurous with your healing and see what happens for you.

Stepping beyond your comfort zone allows you different avenues of healing. Which is sometimes exactly what we need.

Change Your Story

- *Are you open to new ways to heal?*
- *What if you tried something new to heal (that everyone else doubts) and followed your gut?*

- *This week, try three new ways to heal your life (mind, body, soul) and journal the results.*

The forever to-do list

"You cannot live your life to please others. The choice must be yours." – White Queen, Alice in Wonderland

Dissipating the expectation cloud.

Are you one of those people that has a checklist a mile long? Does it all get done? Okay, maybe a few things get done, but you keep adding more? I used to be one of those people. In fact, I used to be *proud* to be one of those people.

Look at my to-do list, look at how much I'm getting done. See my worth. See how valuable I am.

I was the forever to-do list person and told myself it felt so good to check something off that list every day. And, at that point in my life, it did. But that feeling of, *okay now what* always came, and so, I just kept adding things.

I was advised to have only three items on my list each day, and if those three don't get done - that was perfectly fine. But any more than three, and your brain gets overwhelmed.

Be careful how long your list is, it could be lead to system overload.

But first, I had to figure out how how to stop it. I asked myself, was the list benefitting my life? Was it helping me to feel some sort of worth when I laid my head down at night? Was I accomplishing more with the list in hand? Or was I setting myself up for failure? More like the latter if you looked at my lists… I slowly started to realize, that I needed to stop being the forever to-do list person.

So, I started to **cut the to-do list cord.**

First, I put away some of the checklists that were laying around my house. Seems silly, but just getting them out of sight helped. If you see a blank checklist, you're going to want to fill it out — you're only human. That's the first step, is to just stop making the dang list in the first place.

Then, I asked myself where my values stood. What would make me feel like I was accomplishing something, without the list? What did I do daily that would make me feel valuable? Self-care came to the top of my mind, so I started there. Instead of my to-do list being for other people, I started putting myself first. What a concept.

It's not selfish to put yourself first, trust me. It actually helps you be *selfless*.

Then, I started to *feel* into my days instead of having to feel like I *should* be doing something. You ever just robotically go about your day, doing the same things even if they aren't benefitting you, just because you "always did it"? It might be time to kick that one out of bed. Time for a habit audit! Check out *Atomic Habits* by James Clear to conduct your very own habit audit. It's eye-opening, that's for sure.

When I *felt* into my day, I learned that joy was at the top of my list, so I inserted more of that. My new to-do list was looking pretty enticing at this point. I was taking care of myself, and having a little more joy — this could be something I could get used to.

And, lastly, I trusted I would get things done in my own way. I didn't judge myself if things didn't get done (on my list). If we are turning over our days to the Divine, we are ultimately saying, guide me. And, with that weight off your shoulders, you can be guided into some pretty magical things, let me tell you.

So, just for today, could you rip up the to-do list and see what unfolds? Trust me, you will still get things done. You will still mentally check off those things, but that expectation cloud that was following you, will be gone. You can be free to be you.

Your to-do list for the day? Be you.

Change Your Story

- *Do you have a forever to-do list?*
- *Are the things on your list benefiting your life or others? Trim it down to only the necessities and see what unfolds.*
- *Can you go a day without the to-do list? If so, journal it out.*

Remove your labels

"Don't let anyone ever make you feel like you don't deserve what you want." – Patrick Verona, 10 Things I Hate About You

Who am I, *really*?

Do you know those tags on bed sheets that say *DO NOT REMOVE?* I remove them.

In fact, I despise all labels. They put us into boxes, pre-packaged, only to be used with instructions. What does a label really do for us? It defines us. Once we have a definition of who we are, it forces belief systems on us that may not even be ours. So are we just supposed to walk the walk of some tagline someone else wrote?

What if I was just, *Caylin*?

Over the years, I've tried to figure out who I am, as we all do. Even beyond the teenage years, when we think we know everything (and literally know nothing), we are still figuring out who we are. But the tricky part is, everyone and everything has a say in our sphere of influence. We are little identity sponges just walking around soaking up this and that, making it our own.

Even if you're a leader in your space, you're still absorbing energy and ideals from all people and things around you. And as you do this, you're

creating the label of yourself. What does *your* label
say?

Here are a few things that are on my label:

- Loud, outgoing
- Fixed energy
- Stubborn Taurus
- Enneagram Seven
- Manifesting Generator
- Positive energy person
- Enthusiast
- Teacher

None of these labels are necessarily negative.

But, with these labels in place, you feel the pressure
to live up to them. Now, when I head into social
gatherings, I'm the one who has to make sure
everyone is happy—laughing, in a good mood,
having a good time. I'm the one who has to generate
ideas and make things happen. I'm the one who has
to teach people the things that I've learned. I'm the
one who has to consistently show up and do all the
things, otherwise my streak is broken. The streak that
I created, of course.

However, constantly being an enthusiast is draining.
Constantly being outgoing is exhausting. Especially
when you're healing! So, how do you rip your own
labels off and just be the soul that you're meant to
be? **We have to get back to who we truly are.**

Let those labels and expectations fall away, and just
see what happens when you aren't any of those
things.

What's the worst that could happen? You let people down that may have been sucking your energy, anyways? You change how you vibe and things that don't serve you fall away? Or worse yet, you open a door to your soul that brings you joy?

Most of what we think we are, are just the labels and beliefs we put on ourselves or on others. Which sometimes is okay! If those beliefs ring true to us, we are able to be authentic. But, most of the time, they are someone else's beliefs imprinted on us and we make them our own.

The real question is - who are you?

If you were to reach way down into your soul, what is it saying? What does it really feel like to be wholly and authentically you? The truth is, most of us don't know.

But what we can do is *listen*. We can go way back to when we were kids — barefoot, wild, and free — and listen. We can't be the children we once were, but we can listen to label-less freedom.

If you're feeling pressure from labels you put on yourself or others have put on you, sit back and really listen to what they are. Do they need to be removed? Are they guiding you down paths that you don't want to be go? Are you putting yourself in a box that could be restricting your soul? If so, break free!

Find out how to remove those labels so your soul can sing — whatever that means for you.

Once you remove one label, others may fall away as well. Don't be scared (like me) to show others who you really are, it's very freeing. And even if you're not ready to fully remove the labels, just ask yourself if you really believe all the things that people say (or you say) about you. If they don't ring true, try to let them go. It's not going to be easy if those things have clung to you your whole life, but it's all a part of the healing journey.

Fear is the thing we have to face to get through to the other side — the real, non-labeled you.

Change Your Story

- *Do you have labels that you feel may not define who you really are? Write them out.*
- *Are these labels constricting you in any way? Try to remove those that are.*
- *Once you're free of these labels, who remains?*

The energy codes

"Don't you understand? When you give up your dreams, you die." - Nick, Flashdance

It's really just love.

Somewhere along my ~~health journey~~ spiritual awakening, I read *The Energy Codes* by Dr. Sue Morter. As you can probably guess, it has to do with the energy centers of the body — the chakras. I do believe that we have to clear and flush negative energy from these centers in order to stay balanced, and I actively try to do so.

The premise of *The Energy Codes* is that there are systems you can do to clear your energy and get in tune with what your body truly needs. In learning about energy, which is everywhere and is everything, and experiencing Reiki myself, it made sense to me.

There are ways to figure out if your energy is blocked, stagnant, or overactive. Who knew that the chakras could be TOO open? You learn something new every day.

And so, I dove into *The Energy Code* system.

There is an energy-cleansing exercise in this book that I wanted to try. Truth be told, this book is chock full of good information and has been majorly beneficial to my healing journey. But, this one exercise, in particular, I wanted to get into was called, 'Generate love'.

Now, you know I love gratitude and I've been working on opening my heart chakra, as I learned it's the key to all healing. This exercise concentrated on visualizing one person or one thing that made you truly, genuinely happy. Easy, right?

Right off the bat, I was frustrated because I couldn't think of anything or anyone. How sad is that? I couldn't think of one thing or person that made me truly happy without strings or attachments to sadness or past experiences. That one stung a bit.

After a while, I settled on my Dad. He passed in April of 2022. And, while this choice had sadness wrapped around it, it still brought me joy to envision him - his smile, his hugs, his acceptance, and so, I generated love in my heart by pulling out all the things I loved about him (and still do).

To my surprise, it was the smallest of things that lit up my heart center. His little laugh when I told him a silly story, his nicknames for me (Fancy Face), or the times he said the right thing when I didn't know I needed to hear it. It wasn't my graduation or wedding or big monumental moments that I remembered most. It was the small ways that impacted me that came to the surface.

And, my heart lit up like wildfire.

It wouldn't stop. One memory led to another and another. One vision brought me to his house, our lake, riding bikes, sitting out back - it was like a flood of memories just burst through the doors of my heart and flooded all the sadness. Tears came but they were tears of joy and happiness. As you can tell by now, crying is a big part of the healing journey, so you'll have to get used to it.

Out of this heart-center opening experience, I will say that my mind was calm, my body was relaxed and I felt a strong connection to what really matters. Love.

Love is truly the only energy we need to heal.

To be truly loved by someone who doesn't have an opinion of you, who doesn't judge you for who you are trying to be, and who accepts you as you are — flaws and all. Love is the only field of space and time that will make you feel safe. Love is the only place that you can allow your nervous system to take a rest, to stop the survival train. Love is the only place where you can truly be vulnerable and alive.

That's it. It's just love.

There are so many energy centers to cleanse and open, don't get me wrong, but that heart center is a big one. If we can just allow ourselves to feel love and send love, it can break down the blockages in the other areas. This I know to be true.

I encourage you to take some time, close your eyes, lay down, and put your hands on your heart. Ask yourself who or what truly makes you happy without strings or attachments. Don't get frustrated if it doesn't pop right up in your mind (like I did). It may take some time.

After you've settled on it, let it flood you. Let it fully in, and really let that heart center open to all the feelings associated with it. If it's joy, sadness, peacefulness, or sorrow - just let it in. It will always go back to love because that's what the heart does best. Don't judge the feelings that come up, don't guide them, just stay focused on who or what brings you happiness. And, breathe.

You'd be surprised what comes up. When love takes over, nothing can stop it.

Change Your Story

- *When was the last time you thought about something or someone that truly made you happy?*
- *Can you send out a little more love to people today?*
- *What would happen if you opened your heart to yourself daily? Journal it out.*

The emotion code

"Of all the trails in this life, there are some that matter most. It is the trail of a true human being."
Kicking Bird, Dances With Wolves

Wait, I'm carrying the trauma of my ancestors?

Can we carry the pain of our ancestors? Because if we did, that would make a lot of sense for my pain.

Along my journey, I fell into *The Emotion Code* by Dr. Bradley Nelson. I already knew at this point that emotions were a big part of my pain and I was just starting to realize that I needed to process them to feel better. Yes, it took me a while because emotions are painful! I had stuffed them deep down because every time I cried, it was a migraine. And, I didn't want MORE pain, I was already experiencing chronic pain on the daily. A vicious circle. I digress.

This book opened up my eyes to the fact that we could have emotions that were actually stuck inside our bodies — but get this, sometimes they weren't even ours. They could be traumatic experiences and negative emotions that were passed down generationally through our bloodline. Now, that's not even fair!

The Emotion Code is designed to help you alleviate physical discomfort, ease emotional wounds, and restore your relationships. It not only helps you to find out what emotions are stuck but also to release them—which releases your pain.

Think about it like this. Have you had that one stubborn pain that has followed you for months, or even years? I do. I had hip pain that had been with me since I was 25, it kept coming back time and time again. I would get it adjusted by my chiropractor and it would just keep coming back. **That, it turns out, was a stuck emotion**! I learned that we carry trauma in our hips. *The Emotion Code* showed me how to release this.

Of course, I was all in.

Here's how it works. First, find *The Emotion Code* chart (in the book or online). It has the core emotions that we experience in columns and rows. Read through them and allow your brain to simply soak them in, you don't have to memorize them. All the juicy emotions are on there — shame, bitterness, resentment — it goes deep.

Then, ask which emotion needs to be released by conducting a muscle or sway test. This is a natural reaction to yes or no answers that your body provides when asked. For instance, if I asked my body if my name was Caylin, it would sway forward, and that's a yes. You can also have someone perform the hand muscle test (I was shocked, there are several ways to muscle test yourself) by pushing your arm down when you ask for yes or no answers

This is a simple way to find out what emotions are stuck. You can then ask your body, is the emotion that is stuck within me in column A? Or row 2? Each emotion has a correlation to a body part. For instance, anxiety is related to the stomach. Makes sense.

Once you find that trapped emotion, you then take a magnet (any old magnet will do, but I bought a heavy-duty one to really pull them out) and run it from the base of your brain stem to the top of your forehead saying *"I release fear (or insert trapped emotion)"*. Simple.

Well, I went a little overboard.

I released ten emotions on the first day. In the following days, I was crying, low-vibing, a little nauseous, and very emotional. I guess I released too many? There weren't instructions on how many you could release. And, like everything I do, I did too much. But here's the good news.

After this, my pain was slowly dissipating in the hip! I was starting to feel the tightness in my neck fade away. I wasn't as anxious. I really was releasing emotions that were stuck! And, when I learned that there could be stored emotions from my ancestors, I started to ask those to be released too. There was shame from way back in my bloodline that I released…which was strange.

How long had these trapped emotions been in my body?

Regardless, I wanted them out. Come to find out, you can have hundreds of trapped emotions in your body at a time. Get them all out! So, if you are feeling

stagnant, stubborn, or really intense pain, you may
want to try this. And, keep it going. If you're feeling
off, release some emotions. Any time, anywhere. But
leave some recovery time, you may even get a head
cold.

You never know what little thing may get trapped. It
could be a childhood experience or something
someone said at the grocery store - your body keeps
score. Your job is to release it.

And, apparently, you need a magnet to do so.

Change Your Story

- *Do you have stubborn pain that needs to be
  released? Try The Emotion Code!*
- *Are you processing your emotions or holding them
  in? Let them out.*
- *What would happen if you truly felt your feels?
  Journal it all.*

The truth about crystals

"The stones are in me." - Opera Singer, The Fifth Element

Stones aren't going to fix you, but they will help.

Here's a truth bomb. Crystals aren't going to fix you.

There is a common thread in the spiritual world that crystals carry healing powers, which they probably do! They are from the Earth, and they are healing. I believe they have an energy to them that will bring an aspect of healing to you. But, they aren't going to fix you.

Crystals, like the healing journey, are about belief.

We've talked about belief. We know how powerful it is. When you attach belief to something (or someone) your energy flows toward it. Where you place your intention, your energy goes. That in turn, goes for crystals as well. If you get into the crystal world, it can be the rabbit hole of all rabbit holes — and one that can get quite expensive. But it can be worth it if you work the crystals in a way that works for you.

It is said that each crystal has unique attributes that
help in different ways. Much like us. A Rose Quartz,
for example, helps to open your heart to love. But it
also has many different meanings as well, because
it's not just for love. It's multi-faceted, with the
ability to do many different things, if it's placed in
the right places, with the right intentions, at the right
time.

My thought process is that crystals draw in the
energy you need (from the Earth) to accelerate
healing. They aren't meant to be prayed upon like
crucifixes. They are meant as an assist.

**Crystals are the icing on the healing cake, if you
will.**

If I were to say, an Amethyst crystal will heal me and
it doesn't heal me, what have I done? I've fixated on
the fact that this crystal was supposed to heal me,
when in fact, I am the one who has to heal me. The
crystal is just one of the many tools in the healing
process.

**Crystals require both belief and non-attachment to
'work'.**

Having them around is great for your energy. Having
them become a part of your daily life, meditations,
breath work, and when you travel. Think of them as
your little helpers on your healing journey. They
attract all the little things needed to put the pieces in
place on your healing path. And when they are used
in a non-attachment way, they can be very powerful.

Here's how I use crystals (take it or leave it).

I have about thirty various crystals and stones in my life. I have Rose Quartz, Selenite, and Amethyst to draw in love, light, and healing in my bedroom, while I sleep. In my office, I have Black Tourmaline, Selenite, and Blue Lace Agate to attract abundance or to ward off negative energy. In my car, I have Clear Quartz for safety. And, throughout my days, I have random stones that make it into my pockets, purse, or bra for when I feel I need a little something extra. Often, they are Amethyst, Rose, or Clear Quartz. I don't rely on them to heal my broken heart or fix my ailments, I add them to the mix of my healing journey.

And, I'd also like to squash any idea of this being 'witchy'. If you're into crystals, it's not because you're a witch or practicing witchcraft, come on now. It's about drawing energy to you to be able to balance. And, as we've learned, we all need a little help to do so. If we trace them back historically, God made these stones, and they were put here on this Earth to help us. Do with that what you will.

Here's what I found when I have crystals around.

I feel more calm and at peace. I find myself thumbing them, which brings a soothing effect to my mind and nerves. When I look at them, I smile, admiring their beauty — inserting joy to my day. Sometimes, they fall out of my bra and I laugh, bringing me joy. Oh, the funny stories of fallen crystals! (Dr. Sarah Porray, you know what's up.) And, often, they are just there - bringing good energy in, when I don't even realize I need it.

I put a Tiger's Eye under my husband's pillow and watched as his power came back to him in small ways. It was a beautiful thing to behold. I put a Selenite under my pillow and my dreams are vivid and full of messages. I put an Amazonite in my office and watched as my productivity levels soared.

Was it the stones? Nah, it was the energy drawn from them - because the stones are around me, the stones are a representation of me and my energy. It was restoring balance to spaces that were filled with doubt. It was the simple ways they sat, waiting for their turn to bring healing into the world. It was the beauty they drew in, the belief they held, and the power they conjured up.

And, just like I admire our Mother Earth, I admire the stones she birthed for us, all in the name of healing.

Change Your Story

- *Are you a crystal lover? If so, what healing changes have happened to you?*
- *Are you open to using stones to assist your healing journey?*
- *In what ways can you draw positive energy into your home?*

Hypnosis experiment

"It was so good, I almost peed my pants!" - Vivian Ward, Pretty Woman

Are you easily influenced?

As I said, I was willing to try anything to heal. That included hypnosis. If you haven't tried it, it's quite the experience. But only if you're willing to believe that it will work and you have a trusted hypnotherapist. A lot of these experiments are based on really wanting to heal, believing you can heal.

I was down and out in pain. I was drowning in fear of being in pain and I was angry about it all. At the time, I was working at at *Life University*, and I took advantage of their learning development program by enrolling in a Life Coaching class. I remember, it was a Thursday afternoon and I sat in my seat, waiting for the class to begin, same as always. I didn't know there would be a guest speaker.

In walked a hypnotherapist — just another day for her. She talked to us about the power of hypnosis and how it could help you heal for a long time.

I jumped on the skeptic bandwagon. My fellow students had all kinds of questions, and she knocked them out of the park with scientific facts. She even hypnotized someone right in front of us!

And so, my hypnosis interest was born. Right after class, I grabbed her number and scheduled an appointment.

I was able to get in quickly and the day came when I pulled up to the appointment, with apprehension in my heart. All of it felt far too normal to me. The building was normal, the office was much like that of an accountant. I kept waiting for the magic or the mystical, but it was a simple, routine appointment.

She asked me why I was there and I stated, simply, **to get rid of my fear of being in pain.**

After some chit chat, she laid me back in a recliner-style chair and asked me to go to a place in my mind that made me feel safe. I ventured to Murray's Lake, a place in Michigan my family spent summers, a place of many fond memories. And, as I traveled there, she counted backward and snapped her fingers at one, saying you are now asleep. My eyes closed voluntarily. There were no other instructions.

I recall her talking in the background…it was foggy like it was far away. I tried my best to stay focused on being in my "happy place". It was about thirty minutes when she snapped her fingers again and I "woke up". It felt like seconds. I remember her voice and most of what was said, and I kept thinking, *welp, that didn't work.*

When I came to, she said, *"Wow, you're influenced very easily and went under fast."* I didn't know what that

218

meant, so I just nodded. My brain felt blank. My skepticism was taking over but I so desperately wanted to believe this was going to work.

Not much was said, but she thanked me and I was on my way. It was all very simple. I was too naive to ask questions and didn't know the protocol, so I walked out and waited.

And, it hit me right away.

I felt an inexplicable feeling of complete zen. It was like pure ease and relaxation washed over me. Right when I got into my car I felt *different*. I felt calmer. I felt a sense of ease. I looked at the blue sky and it looked more crisp, more clear. It's so hard to explain but I felt brighter. **Lighter**.

I had things to do and I didn't do them. I went and got my toes done instead — something I *never* do. I sat in that pedicure chair and zoned out to the point of pure relaxation. I felt weightless for the first time in years. I kept thinking, what is happening? Is this working? Am I free of pain?

And, the next day I woke up, and I felt *better*. The fear of pain was still there but not as intense. Micro fractions of fears were falling away, which meant I didn't feel as much pain. It didn't happen all at once, it was a slower effect. But it…was working.

I diminished my fear of being in pain by a small amount. I would say it was because I was open and willing to believe it could happen. If I had gone in there with a closed heart and a closed mind, it would not have taken effect. But because I willed it to be true, it was. The power of intention is strong.

Hypnosis may not be for everyone but it was definitely beneficial to me at that point in my life. I will go back.

To this day, I feel that the fear could have taken control over my life. The fear did come back after many years, but I had the tools and support system to help combat it.

My hypnosis experiment results? **If you are willing to be open and to believe, anything is possible.**

Change Your Story

- *Have you ever tried hypnosis? Share your story with me!*
- *Are you open to experimenting with hypnosis to help you heal?*
- *Do you believe that you can heal? Journal it out.*

Shamans, past lives, and light workers, oh my

"I was given a vision that tells us that we belong to something that is greater than ourselves, that we are not... that none of us are alone!" - Eleanor Arroway, Contact

Wait, so I'm a light worker now?

Before you condemn me or stop reading, understand I do this all in the name of healing. I try these things so I know how to help others, through my journey. After all, a scientist wouldn't present a hypothesis without experimenting first, right?

So, here I am, laying down on the front lines, for you —trying all the healing things.

This is my experience talking with a Shaman.

The original connection was through a beautiful friend of mine, Dr. Amy King, who is a Reiki practitioner, chiropractor, and all-around magical soul. We went through the "living on the edge" phase of our lives together, where we partied all night and healed all day. We often joke about how we are lucky to be alive - but we made it, together and now we're swapping Shamans instead of swapping shots.

Speaking to a Shaman was really the one thing I hadn't done, to be honest. I was skeptical, as always, to speak to someone who could be in the scamming biz. But, I digressed because Amy vouched for her light. And I trusted her.

And, so the Shaman session was scheduled. It was a Tuesday morning Zoom call, not at all what you would think. I had no idea what to expect but I logged on like I would a work meeting, and sat there, waiting for my life to change, like always.

Right off the bat, she said my light was so big and bright it almost knocked her back. She said my energy was so beautiful and big that it was clear that I was here to anchor my light and help others. I started to relax a little.

I am very confused about past lives, and past life regression, so I just observe from an open mindset. She told me that I was a warrior and had fought many battles in my previous lives, hence the pain. Huh. I, apparently, was a protector of children — that I was "fighting the good fight" as a healer. Wait, wasn't I healing myself?

She said I need to allow myself to be where I am, and that God (and his angels) see how hard I've been working.

And that my pain is my purpose - of which this book is based.

222

She said my suffering is not for nothing, and that I will be able to help people because I've walked the walk and can talk the talk. I will speak on stages telling my tale (yes, that happened - Janet Jackson microphone and all, more to come on that), and I will be able to intuitively read and help people with breath work (yes, that is happening) and that I am here to not only heal myself (my inner child) but also others. *Well, dang.*

Within the span of two hours, I was able to release my fear of not being safe. I was able to own my space and stop dimming my light, and I started to realize that I needed to step fully into my power. I needed to stop doubting these intuitive hits! I was able to fully trust it and listen to what the Divine was showing me (numbers, signs, synchronicities) and know that they are messages to continue on my path - helping others will help me.

Energy clearing and cleansing would be a big part of what I (and we all) need to do, and understanding my power will come in breadcrumbs (Divine breadcrumbs!). This session even came with instructions on how to do so - for which I was grateful. I love instructions! She also reminded me that I am a badass! I'm a warrior for the good of all people and to never fall short of that. *Woah.*

Since this day, I have opened my eyes to things I didn't know possible. What? You mean I can help someone release their fears too? A Shaman doesn't have to be a trek in the woods in an indecipherable country, shoving plant medicine down your throat, waiving feathers and smoke in your face. It doesn't

have to be what the books say it is. Sometimes it's a
Zoom call on a Tuesday morning. If you're open.

**What you take out of these sessions is yours and
yours alone.**

What I took out of it is that I am powerful, fear
doesn't own me, and I am here for a purpose. You are
that purpose, reader. You are the reason I suffered,
through it all, to share it with you. Sure, I want to
save everyone, I do, but it's one soul at a time — and
all because I took a leap of faith to try something
new. Are you open to doing the same?

Change Your Story

- *Are you open to talking to a trusted Shaman?*
- *Would you be willing to open your healing
  journey to understanding your past?*
- *Are you ready to step into your power? (Yes, you
  are.)*

Tapping through trauma

"When you don't have anything, you don't have anything to lose. Right?" - Samantha, Sixteen Candles

I tried EFT, but I couldn't tap into it.

You ever try something and wonder *am I doing this wrong*? That was my experience with EFT tapping.

Emotional freedom technique (EFT) is an alternative treatment for physical pain and emotional distress. It's also referred to as tapping or psychological acupressure. It focuses on tapping the 12 meridian points of the body to relieve symptoms of a negative experience or emotion.

Gary Craig, therapist and founder of EFT, developed this technique, and he found that a disruption in energy is the cause of all negative emotions and pain. Those that have used this technique believe tapping the body can create a balance in your energy system and treat pain. Though still being researched, EFT tapping has been used to treat people with anxiety and post-traumatic stress disorder (PTSD).

I read *The Healing Code* by Dr. Alex Lloyd and Dr. Ben Johnson, and it goes into great detail about the impact of EFT. So, like always, I was all in.

I read that similar to acupuncture, EFT focuses on the meridian points — or energy hot spots — to restore balance to your energy. **It's believed that restoring this energy balance can relieve symptoms of a negative experience or emotion that may be stuck in your body.**

Here's how it works:

1. First, identify the problem or fear you have. This will be your focal point while you're tapping.

2. Next, set a benchmark level of emotional pain or intensity on a scale from 0 to 10, with 10 being the worst or most difficult.

3. Then, establish a phrase that explains what you're trying to address focusing on two main goals: acknowledgment and acceptance. For example, **"Even though I have this [fear], I completely accept myself."**

4. Now, start tapping on the meridian points in order and recite your focus — side of the hand, top of the head, eyebrow, side of the eye, under the eye, under the nose, chin, collarbones, and under the arm. Repeat this sequence two or three times raising the intensity each time, then rest.

For some reason, nothing was happening. I knew it worked for others, though.

I tried it for a few days. I couldn't find a way to "level my emotional scale" and it felt like I was focusing on the tapping action, not the emotional pain. It was hard to do both - like rubbing your head and patting your stomach. I felt like a drummer, where my hands and my mind had to do different things - and they didn't want to.

I went to do it the next day, and my body didn't want to. Then I watched the *Heal* documentary and saw it in action. I believe that if I went to an EFT professional, I would be able to open up some things that I can't do myself. And perhaps, one day I shall try it.

This is part of the healing journey as well, some things aren't going to resonate with you.

And that's perfectly fine. Don't force it. Be open to it, but don't put pressure on yourself to keep doing something that may not be a fit for your path at that time.

Who knows, I may be able to pick it back up later in life and it will heal some big emotional blockage. My aha EFT moment may come. I'm still open to it.

For those of you who have tried EFT tapping, I want to know all the secrets! Tell me how to be better at it, tell me what I'm missing, because I want to experience emotional freedom, just like anybody else.

Change Your Story

- *Have you tried EFT tapping? If so, how did it help?*
- *Have you had a professional EFT tapping session? Please share your experience if you're willing with me @cbcinked.*
- *Are there tricks to the tapping experience that I'm missing?*

Grounding is not optional anymore

"If you look the right way, you can see that the whole world is a garden." - Mary, The Secret Garden

Earthing is the new ~~black~~ cure.

Who remembers running around barefoot as a kid? We didn't care about anything, we were wild and free, just running through the grass, happy. It was beautiful.

What I've come to learn is that this is called Earthing - quite literally being barefoot and one with the Earth. Essentially, this is how we are meant to be. If you really think about it…humans made shoes - we weren't meant to wear them. We made concrete paths, we made houses to live in. And sure, I am all about living in houses, but we weren't really *meant* to be doing it - as humans.

We were meant to be outside, in nature.

We were meant to live among the trees, breathing real air, feet right in the soil. That's why people feel so good when they garden, go to the beach, or just sit outside. It's our **home**.

Earthing is grounding. How does it work?

229

You guessed it, I dove in wholeheartedly. Here's what I found from the *Earthing* book and documentary.

When you touch the ground with your bare feet or body, the Earth's electrons flow into you. This is called "grounding." The Earth's surface has a limitless supply of mobile electrons that gives the ground we walk on (as well as lakes and oceans) a natural electric charge. When your body touches the ground, it dissipates static electricity and environmental electrical charges through you. At the same time, you receive a charge of energy in the form of free electrons and your body synchronizes with the natural frequencies of the earth. I mean - if that isn't healing, what is?

From the National Library of Medicine:

"Environmental medicine generally addresses environmental factors with a negative impact on human health. However, emerging scientific research has revealed a surprisingly positive and overlooked environmental factor on health: direct physical contact with the vast supply of electrons on the surface of the Earth. Modern lifestyle separates humans from such contact. The research suggests that this disconnect may be a major contributor to physiological dysfunction and unwellness. Reconnection with the Earth's electrons has been found to promote intriguing physiological changes and subjective reports of well-being. Earthing (or grounding) refers to the discovery of benefits — including better sleep and reduced pain — from walking barefoot outside or sitting, working, or sleeping indoors connected to conductive systems that transfer the Earth's electrons from the ground into the body."

230

And it doesn't end there! Remember the term, "tree huggers"? Well, it turns out, tree energy is real and you should hug them. It can heal you.

Deeply rooted in Earth's energy and connecting the universal force of life, trees are the most spiritually evolved living beings on this planet. They are perennially in a meditative state and use a very subtle form of energy as their language. Trees absorb any negative energy and convert it into something useful. The more firmly trees are rooted in the earth, the higher they reach the heavens above. They co-exist with nature and humans and maintain the balance of the living world.

Trees are energy healers, ya'll.

Now I know why I was always sad when I saw trees that had been cut down. I had mad *Ferngully* vibes.

And now, we can bring grounding into our home (because we are still going to live in houses). Unless you want to go live in a hut in the woods, I am not against that at all. Who knows, I may do it one day.

I went a little nuts and bought all the grounding tools for my home. I bought grounding mats for our feet while we watch tv (they look like black mouse pads), I purchased grounding mousepads for our offices while we type, as well as king-sized grounding sheets for our bed and pillow cases.

I also turned the Smart meter on my home back to a dialog meter and turned off 5G on all devices - we don't need any of that. You can also purchase

Shunghite for your home as well to ward off EMF (electric and magnetic fields). And, no SMART devices, sorry *Alexa*.

Even though these are amazing tools, going outside for the real deal is the best for you. So, every day on my lunch break and in the evening, I go out in my tiny foldable chair and park my toes in the grass. Yes, even if it's raining or cold. Because I need to be grounded. And, I am aware that there are fire ants, and the blades of grass are itchy, and it's hot at times…

That's part of health - no one said it would be easy. But it is worth it.

Do you need to be grounded? Yes, the answer is yes.

Change Your Story

- *Do you make time for grounding in your life? If not, can you?*
- *In what ways can you shield yourself from harmful things like EMF in your home?*
- *What would happen if you lived a more grounded life? Journal your story.*

Your home is energy too

"If more people valued home above gold... this world would be a merrier place." - Thorin, The Hobbit: The Battle of the Five Armies

This is your space, make it yours.

Even though we may not choose our home, our home chooses us. I've been through many places I've called "home" in my life, and each one has mattered so much to me.

I've lived in the little red house on the corner, the log cabin in the woods, the dorm room, the rinky-dink apartments, the over-priced condos, and four houses of all shapes and sizes. When it comes to home, I get around.

The beauty of your home is what you make it and who is welcome in it.

When you think of home, what happens inside your body? Does it feel good inside, like freshly baked cookies or the smell of laundry? When you close your eyes, can you picture the sunlight in the kitchen window or the look of the front door? It's all unique to you, but what you do with the energy of your home matters to your healing journey.

I'm sure you've heard of Feng Shui, but I didn't realize just how important it was to the healing process.

Feng Shui, sometimes called Chinese geomancy, is an ancient Chinese traditional practice that claims to use energy forces to harmonize individuals with their surrounding environment. The term Feng Shui means, literally, "wind-water".

By definition, Feng Shui is the practice of arranging pieces in living spaces to create balance with the natural world. The goal is to harness energy forces and establish harmony between you and your environment. Also, it needs to look cool and make sense to you.

I learned some principles that I put into place, that I thought I would share. As with everything in this book, take it or leave it, but make your home yours.

I learned that ideally, you should have a clear line of sight to the door. Also, there is something called a commanding position, an area where you will spend most of your time. Determine this position in the room and then place your bed, desk, or stove in diagonal alignment (if you can). These parts of your house are critical because each represents an essential part of your life. The bed represents you, the desk is your career, and the stove is your nourishment. Cool, huh?

You can go crazy and get a Bagua map, which is a superimposed floor plan of your home, showing the eight areas to work with. Each of the eight areas relates to a different life circumstance, such as family, wealth, or career. And each of these areas has corresponding shapes, colors, seasons, numbers, and earthly elements. At the center of the Bagua — the ninth area — is you, representing your overall wellness.

It can get intense, but I felt out what was right for me and my home. I placed furniture and lighting where my intuition guided me. If it felt wrong, I would walk past it and just feel it. Colors and textures all matter, so allow that to take over when you're decorating your home.

Your goal is to feel good in your space. Your energy will tell you.

Too much clutter can clutter the mind. Get rid of the things that no longer serve you! My advice is to watch the *Minimalism* documentary on Netflix, you will want to get rid of everything. Only hold on to memories or tools that serve you now. The rest can go.

Yes, I had to get rid of the *Super Nintendo* that my Dad bought me when I was nine. It was tough.

And when you have a heavy situation happen in your home, you can clear the energy with some smudge sticks or sage. It may be a little woo-woo for you, but when I did it, I was shocked at how much better I felt after. Sometimes, you just have to clear the air.

Home is what you make it. Make it yours.

Change Your Story

- *What is your home situation like? Can you change it to make it yours?*
- *Do you practice Feng Shui? If not, can you incorporate ways to make your space more enjoyable?*
- *What clutter can you clear from your life? It may be time to clear the air too.*

Yoga truths

"Remember, Red, hope is a good thing, maybe the best of things, and no good thing ever dies." - Andy Dufresne, The Shawshank Redemption

It isn't about the pose, it's about the connection.

All my life, I've been afraid to exercise. I've been scared that if I stretched my muscles or worked out, that I would go out of alignment and be in more pain. And, for most of my life, this was the case. If I did anything extra at all, say, took a jog, my hips, neck, and back would go out of place, causing insane pain throughout my whole body. Alas, I still tried.

The inner me wanted to move.

Every type of workout was followed up with more pain. Eventually, I gave up and realized that I would never get past that boot camp phase of workouts where your body toughens up. It just wasn't in the cards for me.

The only thing I could do - and even that was tough - was walk. I was able to walk it out, and thank heavens for that. I can't tell you how many issues I've solved with a good walk. It's like secret therapy with myself.

I was told by doctors, friends, and family that I probably shouldn't do yoga. Historically speaking, yoga = migraines. I would downward dog myself right into the worst headache of my life. Every time.

I forever wanted to be that yogi, doing a graceful stretch on the mountain top in the sunset. I wanted to be the one who could do a yoga class with her cute mat and then go to work with a coffee in her hand, like the *Sex & the City* ladies.

Yoga is literally stretching the muscles of your body - that's its purpose. Being hyper mobile and inflamed back then, I would stretch and be in immediate pain. But what I didn't realize is that it's more about stretching the mind. And it's also about flow.

It's about connection. It's about breath. It's about freedom.

As I began to heal, I got more confident. I thought to myself - what if I *am* the person who can do yoga? Why can't I be the yogi? So, I would try the videos, the apps and on my own. I slowly started to bend, shape and stretch. But it was all with the shadow of fear at my back. It was all out of the feeling of, I shouldn't be doing this, I could hurt myself. Don't stretch too far, don't do that pose, or that one, definitely not that one. I learned the poses but it wasn't truly learning the art of yoga.

I didn't believe I was able to do it, so my body didn't either.

One day, I just stopped obsessing over it. I stopped thinking that my body was supposed to be

238

something it was not, or my mind was supposed to be doing something it wasn't. I dropped the goal of the ultimate yogi, and I just flowed. It wasn't pretty. It wasn't graceful, but I flowed into whatever my body told me to do. It was simultaneously hard and easy at the same time. I wanted to judge myself, but I didn't. I just allowed my breath to take me from one pose to the next. I allowed my mind to process my thoughts instead of ruminating. I got rid of the "should of" and just leaned into the "what is".

I realized fear was holding me back from yoga.

After six months of 20-minute yoga sessions in the morning, I finally understood what everyone was raving about. It wasn't the actual stretching of the muscles in the poses, it was in between the poses that mattered. It was the coordination with the flow of your breath. It was the connection of the mind. It was centering on what matters most - *you*. It was a dance with your spirit.

And, like all things, I was all in.

I signed up for a package at a local yoga studio and just told myself to take it easy. This would be the first session where I wouldn't end up with a migraine.

I went — open heart, open mind. At the studio, the first thing I saw was a tree that reminded me of one on my Dad's urn and that was enough for me. I was in the right place.

My body was excited, and I noticed it wasn't fueled by fear. I told myself I would be able to do this and I

would do it my way. I'm just a normal girl going to a
yoga class on a Monday morning.

The doors opened and I noticed it was really hot in
there. I wondered if the AC was broken. Regardless, I
went through with it. I sweat and stretched and
sweat and stretched. I felt the yoga glow.

Halfway through the class, I realized it was *really* hot
in there. It finally dawned on me that I had signed up
for a hot yoga session. I would have never in a
million years done this, out of fear. But by not
realizing it, and jumping in (without quitting), I was
able to conquer this fear. Even if I didn't know it, I
was meant to face it. And guess what, I LOVED it.
My body loves the heat! And purging those extra
toxins was double healing power.

I am proud to say that I didn't fall or fart one time. If
you know, you know. I didn't stumble, judge or
ridicule myself. I simply let the movement take me.

I followed up with an Epsom bath and a little extra
CBD, but no migraine. I had broken my historical
record. But now, I wondered, could I keep it up?

As it turns out, it didn't matter if I went to a class or
did it on my own, as long as I did it. So, I did. And to
this day, I have a small Vinyasa-style yoga flow that I
do six days a week, and I love. There are poses that
make me think, some that make me feel, and others
that make me mad. Yes, some poses make me mad.
Hey, you take the good with the bad.

The important thing is that I beat the fear.

And just like all my other fears, it ended up being mist that I walked right through. And not only that, it was joyful. It was something I have done many times since!

Yoga is a beautiful connection to your spirit. It's a wonderful reminder to be present and accepting of all that you are. **It is truly bringing mind body and spirit into harmony.**

And for additional pain management tools (to accompany yoga) here is what I have and use:

- **Foam roller**: A foam roller is a method of self-myofascial release. It's a lightweight, cylindrical tube of compressed foam used for increasing flexibility, reducing soreness, and eliminating muscle knots.
- **Cervical traction unit**: Cervical traction is a treatment for neck pain that involves an apparatus that hangs over your door, lightly pulling your spine to create space between the bones in your cervical vertebrae.
- **Acupressure mat**: An acupressure mat, sometimes called a needle stimulation pad (NSP), is covered with hundreds of plastic points that deliver pressure to various body parts of the body.
- **CBD**: Cannabidiol (CBD) is a cannabinoid compound found in the cannabis plant (non-THC) that produces relaxation and antioxidants (neutralizes destructive oxygen free radicals in cells) for anti-inflammatory properties.
- **Red light:** Red light therapy (RLT) is a treatment of low wavelength red light to

reportedly improve your skin and cellular health.

- **Theragun**: The Theragun is a handheld percussive therapy device that alleviates muscular pain and increases the range of motion in the body.
- **PEA**: Palmitoylethanolamide (PEA) is a supplement used for different types of pain, fibromyalgia, osteoarthritis, multiple sclerosis (MS), carpal tunnel syndrome, autism, and many other conditions.

That's a wrap on pain management tools!

Change Your Story

- *Have you tried something new to move your body?*
- *Would you be open to trying yoga without resistance, judgment or fear?*
- *And what would happen if you dedicated a few moments to your morning for movement?*

Vacuum dancing

"And, David danced before the Lord with all his might... leaping and dancing before the Lord." - Ren MacCormack, Footloose

Sometimes you just have to turn it all the way up.

Whenever I clean, I feel like *Betty Boop* on the old black and white episode where she is picking up after a big party. She's crying because it's so messy. I don't have her *boop-boop-bedoop* powers, but I sure can relate.

I am not a fan of chores. In fact, I am not a fan of doing anything mundane, boring or repetitive. I loathe the constant cleaning - even of myself! Everyday, it's this *again*? Didn't we just do this yesterday?

Daily irritations lead to chronic pain.

You ever just walk around your house, picking things up just grumbling to yourself about how unhappy you are about picking these things up? It's the worst mental train to get on. I was living in this irritable state. I had to break the cleaning blues cycle.

It always seemed to be a big fight inside me. Why was I so mad about having to do ALL the things?

243

Because all I wanted to do was have fun. Is that too much to ask for?

I quickly learned that I had to make peace with cleaning.

So, I asked myself, how can I make this more fun? The only way I thought to do this was to cut loose while cleaning.

What would Betty Boop do?

I made a playlist of all my favorite songs that picked me up. No melancholy tunes here, just all dancy dancy. I added some that I actually new the words to, so I could sing along, and I threw in my headphones. Bruno Mars was up first.

Cleaning was going to be fun whether it liked it or not.

I don't know about you, but I can't fully dance when people are watching. I think someone once remarked about my dancing when I was younger, and I will never really recover, so I often hold myself back. Therein lies the second rule of busting out of the cleaning blues cycle. I needed to be alone.

I clean better when I am free to do it my own crazy way.

When the house is clear and the music is turned all the way up, I can finally bust out in song and dance. Not caring who hears my offbeat singing, not caring who sees my body jiggling around. If you have not literally sang on the top of your lungs while vacuuming, have you even lived?

Cleaning the counters can be enjoyable while belting out Neil Diamond, let me tell you.

Put on a dance mix and let your body do the cleaning. You don't even have to think about it because you are too wrapped up in the music.

Bonus points because you get a workout in too. I've cleaned so hard I was sore the next day. Never underestimate the power of a house cleaning dance party.

The whole point is that you are letting your creative side playyyyy. Now, when I'm driving in my car by myself, I play exactly what I want to hear, and I turn it up! You can catch me singing on the top of my lungs at a stop light and I really won't care. I am enjoying the moment, leave me to my Tina Turner. It's simply the best.

Your body was made to move. It was made to bust out into song (yes, I know our lives are not musicals), it's true. We were made to be joyous and free.

That whole dance like nobody's watching? It's a big healer.

Try it.

Change Your Story

- *Do you allow yourself to cut loose?*

- *How can you make the mundane fun? Do it today!*
- *In what ways can you cut back the things that make you irritable? Journal it out.*

The power and curse of relationships

"You can be my wingman, anytime." - Iceman, Top Gun

People can simultaneously break you down and light you up.

Here's what I've learned about people. They are the lifeblood of our experiences, the reason for our emotions at times, and the connection to the world around us. But they aren't supposed to be the foundation of it. They are a part of the process - not *the* process.

I've had a rough go at relationships over the years. Coming from a divorced family, I learned that people leave. So, I clung on tight to those I cared about. I found someone that made me happy and paid attention to me, and I gave it my all. I often got my heart broken because it's an unhealthy balance of need vs want - I see that now. I was also running from the relationship with myself which I didn't know needed tending.

People are everything. They can build you up or tear you down.

What I learned as I started to guard my heart and open up less, is that people will do whatever they want. They are not like you, they don't think like you, nor have the same experiences as you. You can't expect anything from anyone, and should always be delighted and surprised when something comes your way that is worthwhile. That took me years to figure out.

I put so much investment in people that I lost myself along the way.

I was putting my full happiness into my relationships. If my relationships weren't healthy, I wasn't happy. If my boyfriend, husband, best friend, or sister wasn't happy with me - I wasn't happy. Period. I didn't want any conflict of any sort, I was never good at handling it. I wanted everyone to be happy all the time. And, I wanted to be at the core root of that.

Cue, people pleasing.

I get it, and I know it's a popular theme people are catching on to. I just didn't know how to turn it off. I didn't know when to say no. I didn't want people to not like me. It mattered so much to me to have their love, their respect, their God-knows-what. I just needed something. I needed to stand on my own two feet without anyone helping me, and man, that was hard.

When my Dad died, I finally woke up to the fact that people are going to leave, and that was okay. It's perfectly fine to lose a friend that was toxic to your growth or to have someone walk out of your life that was causing you pain, or a door that was closed in your face to allow room for something better. It's okay to not have closure from that argument, or that a person is talking poorly behind your back. It's okay because **it's all a reflection of them**.

I started to let go of this and the need to make others happy. I really needed to be happy with myself and I had no idea how to do that because my body and mind had betrayed me for years. My relationships were jaded from the past. It took me months of soul-searching to finally be okay with just me. I stopped putting stock in others for my happiness and I was finally okay to be alone with myself and actually be content.

And, just like that, space opened up and my spiritual community found me.

Enter: Divine breadcrumb trail. From my first visit to my sound healer, Brandee, to an invitation to the Circle of Light gatherings, it was meeting person after person after person filled with nothing but love and light. I had asked for new souls to enter my life that would help me through this healing journey, and God did not disappoint.

The community that found me took me in as one of their own and really saw me for me. There was no judgment, no eggshells to walk on, no competition or inauthenticity. It was raw and real and beautiful. More importantly, I didn't rely on them for happiness. They were a part of my own circle of healing.

We've since hosted healing events, weekend-long retreats, and had magical moments together that are helping to heal others. As soon as I let go of those toxic relationships and made peace with myself, it made space for these beautiful souls to enter my life. And, I am forever grateful for their love, support, and grace. Each one of their stories lifts me up and makes me feel I am in the right place. That's what a true community does.

When the time is right, your tribe will find you.

Change Your Story

- *How do your relationships impact your life?*
- *Have you made your relationship with yourself a priority?*
- *Do you have a community where you feel you can be your authentic self? If not, can you make space for them to find you?*

Water is life

"Water is powerful. It can wash away earth, put out fire, and even destroy iron." - Mameha, Memoirs of a Geisha

I get why I wanted to be a mermaid now.

Water may be one of the biggest tools in this healing journey. You may be thinking, *sure, Caylin, we all know we need to drink water to survive.* It's so much more than that.

Water is life, it is Source, it is literally everything.

When I was young, we used to have jugs of cold, fresh water just sitting around and it was the most refreshing thing to take that first sip. When we drink water, we don't realize all that it's doing for us. We take it for granted, just like the air we breathe.

It wasn't until I was much older (and after many years of dehydration) that I realized that water is so much more to me and a big part of this hearing journey. Water is the way of so many things if you really think about it.

We are born of water, we are made of water and we need water to survive. It's one of those magical things that comes in all forms and no matter which

251

one it is, they are all good for us. **We are, quite literally, one with water.**

After I learned about the importance of filters, I purchased a *Berkey* water filtration system. It was expensive and I saved up for it, like a kid wanting a new toy. Water isn't what it used to be and the systems that run our pipelines are not quite filtering what we need for our bodies. I shudder to think of the chemicals that I have consumed over the years, but I digress.

Step one, filter your water.

Step two, get near water in some form. The healing powers of the ocean far surpass many healing modalities and are quite possibly on the top of my list. It's scientifically proven that when you are around bodies of water (even retention ponds), you physically and emotionally calm down. It triggers a relaxation throughout your entire body that, well, is much needed honestly. We are going so fast, our minds never stop, and when we look at water, we are simply vibing with its energy.

The feelings I've experienced while staring out at the ocean or a lake are one of a kind. It's like the water opens up a side of you that you need to listen to. It allows you to process things differently. And, things become clearer - even if it's painful.

Want to heal? Get to water.

Step three, become one with water. I cannot tell you the immense relief from simply taking a bath. If you can get yourself in water, that's sometimes all you need. A shower, a sprinkler, a hot tub, a pool, or a bath - just get your body in water. It is healing for your body to feel weightless, buoyant against the harshness of the world. It's cathartic to let yourself be free of the weight of life around you. Why do you think little girls wanted to become mermaids? It's so freeing to be in water, like you are one with nature.

I just learned of something called a sacred bath. A sacred bath is what you make it, there are no protocols or proper tools. I realized I wasn't making my bath time special, as I was using it solely as a healing modality. I was in pain and the hot water made my body feel better. But it became more than that. It became time to breathe, be, and pray. My sacred bath now consists of lavender candles, sage smudge sticks, sound healing music, and no technology. It became a space for me to process, express and actually open up. I didn't check my texts, or open a book, I just breathed with my body, in the water. What came up, went into the water.

There have been many baths filled with gut-wrenching tears, truthful conversations with myself, and epic realizations. I'm not sure if the water draws it out, or it was just the way it was meant to be.

You want real healing? Create a sacred bath.

Whether you're a water lover or not, make it a part of your healing journey in a new way. Prioritizing water to drink, be with, or be in is now important to true healing. Water has energy and if you speak into it, it can carry great things. This is all new to me, but it makes sense as we are one with nature.

Water is life. You are life.

Change Your Story

- *Do you prioritize quality water in your life?*
- *How do you feel when you are in or around water? Are you allowing it to heal you?*
- *What if you made a scared bath (and time for yourself) weekly? Journal it out.*

Cutting the cord

Sometimes you have to sever ties.

Forgiveness is essential to the healing journey. This I know to be true. Forgiving yourself and others is a turning point that allows your heart to open. But, and this is a *big* but, there comes a point in life where you must make a decision. If people have hurt you, there is no resolution, and they are not willing to change or the hurt is far too deep, is it time to cut the cord?

Sometimes it can get to be too much. You're attaching your health to this pain and you can't heal. For instance, do you catch yourself ruminating over what you could have said or done differently? Does your heart ever ache so badly that you wish you never had that experience? Or perhaps you were hurt so badly that you feel it may make a permanent mark on your soul. This needs healing.

Enter cord-cutting.

This concept is one that I used frequently in my healing. Here's what I learned. We're all energetically connected to every person that walks into and out of our lives. Some of these connections are fleeting and weak; others are binding and strong. Thankfully, I learned that we have control over our energetic ties.

We have the power to say if someone can take our power.

Cord-cutting is the process of severing our energetic connections to people, fears, or experiences that are hindering our healing and growth. It is essential to let go as it may be weighing you down and holding you back. These bonds can hinder your energy and keep you stuck in old thoughts and patterns. And, they definitely were for me.

When we cut the cords of these people and experiences, we are opening space for mental clarity. We are improving our physical health, releasing pain, opening passageways in our energetic field, and healing our relationship with ourself and others.

You can search for cord-cutting ceremonies anywhere and there will be everything from blowing out a candle to physically cutting yarn from around your ankles. My advice is to turn inward and listen to what your heart is saying. Are you ready to let this person or experience go? If so, it's time to cut the cord.

Here's what I did to cut the cords of the people in my life that had hurt me beyond repair.

I drew a bath. I dressed up the bath a bit with a few extra candles. I diffused some lavender essential oil and dimmed the lights. I made sure I wasn't going to be interrupted. I pulled a Rose Quartz heart-shaped stone my sister had gotten me because it made me feel loved, and set it out on the ledge. I tuned into soft meditation music, with beach wave sounds behind it because the sea speaks to me.

I sat in the bath for a while and breathed into my emotions. I *really* felt them. I allowed them to really hurt. Tears came and went. Then I began to imagine a cord from my heart to this person. I just sat with this for a while and asked myself how it felt. I leaned in to all the experiences with them and how it made me feel.

There was a cord running from my heart to theirs, strong in my mind.

Then I envisioned that I cut the cord of this bond and let it fall far away. I envisioned the person fading into the mist. No longer able to hurt me. I imagined all of the ways I could feel now that I was free. I no longer had to hold on to that pain. I no longer had to give my power away.

I was free.

I breathed through this feeling of relief and allowed myself peace with it. I allowed whatever to come up to come. I allowed whatever to go, to go.

And, then — the hardest part of all — I put my hands to my heart and I *thanked* them. I thanked them for showing me what I did not deserve. I thanked them for showing me how to set boundaries. I thanked them for showing me how I could grow from this. I thanked them for the suffering because it allowed me to face my shadow self and cut the cords of my past.

Talk about intense.

From that day on, I still think about that person but it doesn't control me. It wasn't stringing me along out of hurt. It was a mix of sadness for their loss and sending them love. It was as if it was a distant memory that now lived far away in my mind, instead of front and center. I made space.

Sometimes, you just have to sever the ties so you can grow.

Change Your Story

- *Do you have hurtful energetic connections to people or experiences that needs to be cut?*
- *What would happen if you cut the ties of connection to this pain?*
- *Are you willing to conduct a cord-cutting ceremony to sever the hurtful ties in your life? Journal it out.*

Stepping into your power

"We will not go quietly into the night! We will not vanish without a fight! We're going to live on. We're going to survive! This is our Independence Day!" - President Thomas J. Whitmore, Independence Day

This is my fight song.

Through all this pain and suffering, there came enlightenment. Finally, a silver lining. I changed my story. And, you can too.

Fast forward to the present, where I write these last words with gratitude in my heart. My body is strong, my mind is clear, my heart is open. With each day that passes, I learn something new about my abilities, my strength, and my resolve. I no longer look at the world as a fearful place. I wake each morning with love and kindness in my heart.

My pain levels went from 90% down to 10% when I changed my story.

Don't get me wrong, every moment is not serene and peaceful. In fact, it's actually the same as before, I am the one who has changed. There are still roadblocks, challenges and rips in the healing fabric, however, I simply changed how I react to them. This is the beauty of turning inward.

Anger, fear and anxiety don't own me anymore.

The toxic relationships still live in my past. I just don't live there anymore. The pain is a distant memory. The dishes are still there. And, this is the beautiful unfoldment. The day I thanked my body for all the pain was the day it all turned around. When you begin to surrender and trust, you slowly become who you were meant to be, and you realize that there is no one else you'd rather be.

I was led, by Divine breadcrumbs, to a meditation certification, which led to a breath work certification. I didn't even think twice about it. All because I was meant to help others. I never knew were it would lead.

The day I guided my first meditation it sank in. I looked around the room at the people with closed eyes and hands on their hearts, breathing, and I felt a swelling of pure gratefulness in my whole body. I was once in their shoes, searching for answers, doubting everything. I am now on the other side of fear, helping others to see the light.

Not to mention I had a sweet Janet Jackson wireless microphone on my ear and a spotlight on me - that felt pretty powerful.

I did it. I found my purpose in my pain.

Not only that, but I've passed it on to my family and friends. As you know, family is the hardest to help, so that took quite a bit. But once I spoke my truth about healing, I was able to open doors for healing others. Through breath work and emotional release, I've been able to help my nephew past his internal challenges. Through diet and supplement changes, I've been able to help my family and friends with their hurdles. Through intuitive messages, I've been able to help my closest friends, clients, and strangers. And, it's all because I believed. I changed.

Because I am not my diagnosis.

As I guide others in mindful meditation and breath work, I am anchoring my light out into the world, which will then help others to anchor theirs as well. Each time we heal, we're healing the entire collective. We are all one conscious collective, and we're all in this together. Healing is the only way we will survive this thing called life.

The truth is, we are all superheroes. We all have the power to change our story. We just have to tap into who we really are, what we are capable of and the tools needed to get there. I will never stop trying, never stop learning — no matter what health issue comes my way. I refuse to stop fighting.

If I have another story to change, you better believe that I will.

Change Your Story

- *Do you have a story to change in your life?*
- *In what small ways can you make those changes for the better?*

- *Are you willing to help others change their story? Let me know!*

"Goonies never say die!" - Mikey, The Goonies

Change Your Story

More by Caylin Brie White:

Goldify
Sliced Time